Yeah, No.
Not Happening.

Also by Karen Karbo

Fiction

Trespassers Welcome Here

The Diamond Lane

Motherhood Made a Man Out of Me

Nonfiction

Generation Ex: Tales from the Second Wives Club

The Stuff of Life: A Daughter's Memoir

How to Hepburn: Lessons on Living from Kate the Great

The Gospel According to Coco Chanel: Life Lessons from the World's Most Elegant Woman

How Georgia Became O'Keeffe: Lessons on the Art of Living

Julia Child Rules: Lessons on Savoring Life

In Praise of Difficult Women: Life Lessons from 29 Heroines Who Dared to Break the Rules

For Younger Readers

Minerva Clark Gets a Clue

Minerva Clark Goes to the Dogs

Minerva Clark Gives Up the Ghost

Yeah, No.
Not Happening.

How I Found Happiness Swearing Off
Self-Improvement and Saying F*ck It All—
and How You Can Too

Karen Karbo

HARPER WAVE

An Imprint of HarperCollins*Publishers*

HarperCollins books may be purchased for educational, business, or sales promotional use. For information, please email the Special Markets Department at SPsales@harpercollins.com.

FIRST EDITION

Library of Congress Cataloging-in-Publication Data has been applied for.

ISBN 978-0-06-294554-9

20 21 22 23 24 LSC 10 9 8 7 6 5 4 3 2 1

For Kathy, who taught me how to enjoy life,
and swearing

An edited excerpt from my morning pages, before I swore off self-improvement.

Today, I should eat more leafy greens. I should have a smoothie at lunch instead of a sandwich. Dave's Killer Bread is organic, non-GMO, verified whole grain, but it's still bread. I read somewhere that even if you don't have a gluten thing, wheat fucks up your brain or gives you bloat, one of the two. I should be more mindful of my gut health in general. I do chug a Lemon Ginger KeVita Sparkling Probiotic Drink instead of the usual Diet Pepsi with my daily afternoon bowl of buttered popcorn. That's got to be an improvement. But I should really find out what probiotics are. Are they the opposite of antibiotics?

I should be a more adventurous eater in general. It took me a long time to get on the quinoa bandwagon, because I couldn't pronounce it and was too embarrassed to ask. Maybe farro (pronounced like *pharaoh*, yes?).

I know they say you should meditate first thing in the morning, but first thing in the morning I haven't had enough time to be completely disappointed in myself or the day yet, so it seems like a waste of time. I should really do the twenty-minute Headspace meditation instead of the ten-minute slacker option. I should do it twice a day, like David Lynch and other cool creative people. David Lynch has been meditating every day for nine hundred years. Without Headspace.

I should really wear my Fitbit. I threw it in my jewelry basket on the bathroom counter because I was sick of it beeping at me all the time. Also, I couldn't shake the feeling of being a lab rat. On the days I didn't make my 7,500 steps (already down from the required 10,000 steps), I felt like a failure. I figured out if I waved my arms around a lot it thought I was walking, but who am I kidding? Myself. I'm kidding myself. I should stop doing that, even though it seems like self-delusion is a key component to self-improvement.

Contents

Introduction: Hello You

To be yourself in a world that is constantly trying to make you something else is the greatest accomplishment.

—Ralph Waldo Emerson

Women are the self-improvers of the world. Those famous Paleolithic cave paintings in France and Spain? Created not by bison hunters dabbling in self-expression, as originally supposed, but by cave women inventing interior design. *This cave is a dump! Let's add a few stick animals and handprints to liven up the place.* Then came the wealthy ladies of ancient Egypt, early adopters of makeup and the practice of spending a fortune on it. We have Nefertiti and Cleopatra to thank for black eyeliner, blue eye shadow, and the classic red lippy. Eleanor of Aquitaine, queen of France, then England, during the twelfth century, was also queen of self-betterment: she could read and speak Latin; sing and play the harp; weave, spin, sew, and whip up a fetching needlepoint pillow; identify the constellations; ride, hunt, and hawk. She literally and figuratively *ruled*.

Fast-forward to the twenty-first century, where this lovely feminine impulse to beautify and improve self and surroundings has evolved into a nutty, near-religious pursuit of perfection. We ladies of late-stage capitalism spend our days chasing the ever-receding mirage of our so-called best selves, existing in a continuous state of telling ourselves we'll do better, be better, and always be thinner or fitter.[*]

We drift off to sleep at night knowing that in the morning we must awake naturally, without the alarm. We must think positive thoughts as we arise in the dark, slip into our flattering athleisure ensemble, then knock out a ninety-minute workout that would bring a Navy SEAL to their knees. We must then meditate, read, and journal. We must say our affirmations. We must make sure the kids have their homework and correct uniforms or instruments for their extracurriculars. We must pack nourishing lunches for them, being careful not to include anything that will cause them to be ostracized from their usual table. We must not lose our temper, but rather practice gratitude, as we try to shove something semi-healthy into their ungrateful little maws, then chauffeur them to school as they stare at their devices. All this before our own breakfast, which

---

[*] No woman on earth has said, "As soon as I can feel my thighs rub together, I'm going swimsuit shopping."

usually involves a fibrous green avoided even by the starving hordes of yesteryear.

The rigors of modern self-improvement are exhausting. One *Huffington Post* piece about cramming some self-improvery into your life involved a "6:00 a.m. outdoor boot camp" followed by a parsley protein shake. Inc.com offers "50 Ideas to Help You Design Your Morning Routine," including making a video log upon waking, working on a side hustle or business idea, learning one to three new things, taking a cold shower after doing a complicated breathing routine that looks as if it might make you pass out, and reviewing your previous day's spending.

Are you a mom? Are you trying to get pregnant? Are you a millennial trying to figure out adulting? Are you trying to crush it in your career? Are you an artist? Massage therapist? Head of HR? Are you a survivor? Empty nester? Church lady? Every demographic brings with it a list of impossible-to-achieve nonsense to which women are expected to aspire. Meanwhile, life is passing us by.

I am *done*, reader. Done viewing myself as a permanent fixer-upper. Done feeling that I'm always supposed to be doing something to better myself, then feeling guilty about being too lazy to commit to the latest self-improvement regimen, or, conversely, if I *have* committed to said regimen, feeling as if I'm not doing it enough or with the proper pure and holy mindset. I'm done feeling bad that I don't live in a perpetual state of red-carpet readiness, even though there is no red carpet to walk, and done feeling that it's my fault I can't stop time, thereby remaining an eternal tousled-hair beauty clad in an oversize cashmere sweater and no pants,* sipping tea from an artisanal mug by a fire made by a man who pulls down seven figures.

Done done done.

So, I decided to swear off self-improvement. A lifetime of striving and struggling to improve myself hadn't yielded much other than frustration and self-loathing. I was fit enough, fifteen or so pounds overweight, a domestic disaster, an avid reader, a rescuer of dogs, a good friend. I was no stranger to an apple or a green salad. I got enough sleep and flossed regularly. I didn't smoke. That was going to have to be good enough.

But I was afraid. Would I instantly transform into a troll under a bridge if I gave up face serum? Would I become the laziest sloth in Slothville if I made yeah, no, not happening my regular morning routine? Would my husband leave me if my glutes and abs stayed exactly as firm as they are this minute, adjusting for age? I worried that I would gain weight, even though the last time I said fuck it all to dieting, I lost a few pounds, just as the people who beat the drum for that approach to eating always promise. The worst thing that would happen, that did happen, is that I got real about who I was, what I enjoy, and how much I just don't give a fuck about all the self-improvery foisted on women.

---

* Why is this even a thing? Every winter, right about the time eggnog lattes return to the Starbucks menu board, we are treated to glossy photos online and in magazines of hot women wandering around in a sweater with no pants.

So far, I'm less anxious, and less worried that whatever I'm doing I should be doing something else, and have more time to devote to stuff I'm interested in. Like singing karaoke while slightly hammered, slinging around my awful high school French, and napping. My blood pressure has gone down. And I've lost seven pounds, even though I said yeah, no, not happening to kale. I hate that shit. It's a decorative winter shrub and should go back to where it came from.

I've written this book to urge you to join me in the radical act of swearing off the endless quest for self-improvement. To stop thinking wistfully and magically that tomorrow you will start the diet, the challenge, the program, the method. To bid a respectful adieu to your imaginary best self, the one you will always fail to inhabit.

A few things before we get started:

Learning to say yeah, no, not happening isn't about giving up on yourself, or health, or beauty. It's about reclaiming your common sense and your confidence that you know what works for you and what doesn't. It's not about settling for a lesser life, but experiencing *more*, because you're no longer captive to the ridiculous, ever-shifting demands pressed upon women in the modern world, most of which are expensive, time-consuming, not very much fun, and fucking lame. It's about standing up for yourself, to yourself, and to the world.

Saying yeah, no, not happening makes space for who we are this minute. This book isn't a self-improvement program disguised as an anti-self-improvement manifesto. Regardless of where we are in life, we've all absorbed messages from our mothers, our peers, and mass consumer culture about what it means to be a successful female. We are who we are, right here, right now.

In addition to demonstrating how to say yeah, no, not happening going forward, I will encourage you to give yourself a break for long-established habits that may technically be considered self-improvement. Some of the ways in which we are pressed into improving ourselves and being "better" women *do* resonate with us. We can't help it, nor do we want to help it. We like our red lipstick. It's part of who we are. When we say "no more" to new self-improvement schemes, we are saying it from where we are this minute. Part of chucking the impulse to self-improvery also involves swearing off perfectionism and celebrating our inconsistencies and contradictory natures. It means understanding that there is beauty in complexity.

Additionally, it bears noting that I come from a place of considerable privilege. I am a cisgender, heteronormative, white, middle-aged woman with a college degree, and this is the only experience I can address with any authority. That said, all women living in a capitalist consumer culture are subjected to the message that they're not good enough and coerced into spending whatever resources they possess to try to improve themselves, and I'm hopeful that my observations aren't merely of interest to my white sisters of the (vanishing) middle class, although I can't guarantee this will be the case.

The politics of self-improvement in the digital age, and the way in which women are effectively hobbled by their inward focus on bettering themselves, deserves a book of its own. Here, I'm focused on how self-improvement affects us personally, in the belief that if we're able to say fuck it all and swear off a portion of the self-improvery nonsense thrust in our direction, we would have the time and space to look up and out at the world. The amount of time, energy, and money women of privilege spend on self-improvement rivals the sun as a power source. Imagine what the world would be like if we directed even half of that toward lifting up other women and doing our bit to save democracy, not to mention the planet.

In the end, your most basic task in life should be to occupy the you of you. I'm not going to use the word *celebrate*. It's overused and brings with it the expectation of treating yourself to something ridiculous and expensive, then overposting it on social media. Occupying the you of you is not just good enough, it's *good*.

A beating heart.

A human soul.

A character and personality like a beech tree—you know the ones I mean, blown into crazy shapes to accommodate the elements. You are flawed. You are wondrous. Why try to square the corners? Why iron out the creases? Why fall for the wisdom of someone else who doesn't know you, who's just trying to make a buck?

There are over a thousand known varieties of bananas in the world. The one we buy in the store is called the Cavendish. Think of it. More than nine hundred ninety-nine other kinds of bananas, but what winds up in our lunch sacks and fruit salads and in the sad buffet at the Holiday Inn Express? The Cavendish.

We are pressed into thinking we all must be the Cavendish. From outside and in, we get the message dozens of times a day. We must be slim and trim and grateful, and leafy green–eating and journal-keeping and productive geniuses of decluttering and hygge (hand-knitted slippers, cozy fire, home-baked gluten-free cookies, bingeing prestige shows on Netflix), posting wacky pictures of our rescue pets (guilty as charged), and endlessly prepping for the next trendy "challenge."

Let's say yeah, no, not happening to all of it. Let us be those other bananas.

Swearing off self-improvement means swearing off a life of overthinking, chronic rumination, and self-doubt. It means trusting yourself and your own judgment. The more we do this, the more our confidence grows. We begin to know who we are, what's worth our time and what isn't. We begin to feel more at ease owning, cherishing, and strutting our impeccable, imperfect selves.

It's sobering that even now being who we are is a rebellious act.

PART I

CHAPTER 1

Today Is the Day

And, like all the best quests, in the end, I did it all for a girl: me.
—Caitlin Moran, *How to Build a Girl*

On March 3, 1979, I began a diet in which I lost twenty pounds. On April 19, 1988, I began a diet in which I lost twenty-three pounds. On June 13, 1998, I began a diet in which I lost thirty-seven pounds. I know these dates by heart. I recall them much easier than I do any other important dates, save my daughter's birthday. Graduations, wedding anniversaries, publication dates, that one Thanksgiving when no one drank too much and got sad—all less memorable than a trio of days a decade apart when I started a diet and stuck with it. Pathetic.

More pathetic still: I haven't been able to stick to a diet, rebranded in our times as a clean-eating plan, for twenty-two years, but that doesn't stop me from telling myself on the first day of the month (also the fifteenth, and, if I'm going to be honest, every Monday) *today* is the day. Today is the day I am going to get back on track. Today is the day I am going to become more productive, more creative, more organized, and less curmudgeonly. I'm going to become a more loving, sexy, and agreeable partner, a better mom, and a more supportive and understanding friend. And thinner. Every time I've decided to do something to improve myself, losing weight is always part of the plan. Being thinner is the crisp white wine of self-improvery; it pairs well with everything.

I haven't really been trying to lose weight since the days when carbs were good and Entenmann's Fat-Free Danish was considered healthier than an avocado. Even so, upon awaking on the first or fifteenth of the month, and every Monday morning, I've told myself today was the day. It had become a habit, like hanging my clothes according to color and swishing after flossing with the original Listerine, the one that tastes like something used to clean an operating room. Even as I told myself today was the day, I was under no illusion that I would do anything but fail, so I got it over with as quickly as possible, driving three blocks to my favorite breakfast spot for a waffle, then returning home to waste the morning online. The irony is this: if today was *not* the day I was getting back on track, I would have drifted into my regular morning, not-completely-unhealthy routine—peanut butter on whole grain toast for breakfast, then a run around the neighborhood until I couldn't stand the boredom, generally about twenty-five minutes.

If you met me, I'm confident you wouldn't imagine I was this deranged. You might have the same impression of me that

4

I have of Janet, a business coach and consultant who also hosts a podcast for entrepreneurial women. Janet is one of those soft-spoken kick-ass women, with a pretty smile and warm demeanor. Her mission is to cure women of the urge to apologize for their ambition and to help them to learn "how to CEO." There are plenty of women working in middle management, but corporate leadership remains less than 10 percent female. Janet's job is to help women over that hurdle. She's passionate in her belief that women have been sold a load of crap, that society has convinced us that success and happiness rely on constantly working to improve ourselves, rather than on the acquisition of practical skills. "Take self-care. It's not massages and mani-pedis but learning how to say no to things you don't want to do. That's really taking care of yourself," she says.

I called her up. I figured, if anyone was immune to the compulsive urge to improve herself, it would be Janet. When I asked her secret, she dropped her phone. I could hear her laughing as she picked it up. Janet, it turned out, was just as imprisoned by self-improvement as anyone else. She was in a regular panic about meal planning. Before she started her job, every meal had four colors. Now it was frozen pizza in the oven, over which she experienced heart palpitation–inducing guilt. Her "shoulding" was off the charts. She should be getting more exercise, tracking her steps, journaling. Every night she said she spent at least an hour online looking for programs that would help her create balance, or a "magic tool" that would help her become a better wife, mom, sister, friend, and businesswoman. "I never feel optimistic about improving myself," she said, "because when it comes to self-improvement, there is always a better better beyond better. There is always something more we can do. There are always more steps we can take."

As I write this, Roxane Gay tweeted: "I am tired of self-improvement. I have done so many terrible difficult things this year. I just want to be trash for a while and have that be okay."

I'm in full agreement. Can't we just be who we are and have that be okay? I would literally rather have a minor medical procedure, with its attendant drama and excellent drugs, followed by the satisfaction of watching my wound heal, than get back on track, choose kale over spinach (these days, opting for spinach is like eating a Twinkie), read more literature and fewer cheesy thrillers, listen to jazz or at least something more culturally enriching than the Spotify Workout Twerkout Playlist, get more and better exercise, meditate my face off, be more mindful, learn to love cooking (knowing full well this will never happen), give back to the community (or more to the community: I already volunteered—but not enough!), become a better listener even when he wants to talk about motorcycle parts, or tackle my to-do list (i.e., make a to-do list).

I have wept more than once at the ridiculousness of it all. At the waste of time. At the endless self-recrimination. And yet, to stop trying to improve myself was synonymous with failure. To be a good woman in the twenty-first century is to be a woman on a continuous quest to be better. To be trash for a while—

that is, a woman who doesn't care to improve herself—is never okay. And somehow, it's never okay to be never okay.

The eternal quest for self-improvement is a self-generating self-doubt machine, and yet we are still seduced by the bogus come-on of people like self-described #1 life and business strategist Tony Robbins, who assures his own job security by preaching "constant, never-ending improvement," confirming that we have as much of a chance of reaching our self-improvement goals as we do of coming to the end of our Facebook newsfeeds.

Self-improvement is a thriving, multigazillion-dollar-a-year industry. Why is that? If all the programs, plans, systems, treatments, or magical cornerstones transformed your life, fixing whatever you believed was wrong with you, wouldn't it be a one-and-done sort of thing? Or maybe more like painting the living room, which happens once a decade, instead of an ongoing slog (otherwise known as a sacred daily practice)? If all this stuff worked, wouldn't self-improvement be a multi*thousand*-dollar-a-year industry? Wouldn't a new thing come along that we would feel compelled to fix—as I write, the health of our gut flora is causing a lot of insomnia across the land—and we would fix it, and then we could go on and we could turn our gaze outward and enjoy being human beings in a beautiful, endlessly surprising world?

While we're on the topic, gut flora is a perfect example of how the knee-jerk compulsion to improve ourselves operates. Until recently, no one but your cousin the gastroenterologist even knew gut flora existed. If we thought about gut flora at all, we assumed she was the lead singer of a punk band.

Over the past decade microbiologists have discovered that our gastric microbes aren't just lounging around our GI tract, waiting to digest the next burrito that comes down the chute, but have an active role in our overall health, *including* our mental health. Gut flora may play a part in our moods, specifically depression. This is fascinating, but notice the word *may*. Research is pointing to this development, but more studies still need to be done, and those studies take years. Science moves slow. Corporations, hoping to capitalize on a flurry of headlines, move fast. No sooner is #gutflora trending on social media than Whole Foods has devoted an entire aisle to gut flora–health-improving supplements and pricey gut flora–balancing beverages. Chances are, unless you've participated in the American Gut Project (where, for $69 and enough chutzpah to poop into a vial and pop it in the mail), you don't even know what's in there. And yet, there you are (there I am), doing your bit to improve it.[*]

It's a familiar cycle: we are made to feel uncertain about something to which we'd never given a thought. We madly google it, absorb conflicting and probably dubious information, fret a little more, and narrow our search to "experts" or our most trusted (usually for no good reason other than we like their pictures) social media gurus. To be clear, it's not as if so-

---

[*] All this said, KeVita's Lemon Ginger Sparkling Probiotic Drink is delish.

cial media gurus are *all* peddling snake oil—some may have a good tip or two—it's believing they know *more* about you than you do about yourself that trains you to doubt yourself. You stop trusting your own judgment. As if you've never learned a life lesson on your own. Our own wisdom comes to seem suspect, as does our ability to decide whether what we're feeling uncertain about is even a problem.

Before I started saying yeah, no, not happening, I came across something about the rise of social anxiety. At the time, I was deeply into avoiding parties. I did that annoying thing where I would optimistically accept an Evite, hoping that in six weeks' time I would somehow be miraculously transformed into a person who would enjoy a costume karaoke party and pig roast. That has never happened once. Yet every time I clicked on YES, followed by the writing of a gushy, insincere note ("We are so looking forward to sushi 'n charades at your place with your in-laws! Can't wait! This is going to be soooo much fun!!!"), I tried to believe it would be fun because clearly other people, other women, thought these parties were a blast. Then I came upon the social anxiety piece and felt relieved. If I suffered from social anxiety, I could fix it. I could improve myself rather than do the hard work of accepting that I was a slightly introverted curmudgeon with a low tolerance for kicky gatherings.

It would be one thing if our self-doubt was limited to managing our gut flora health and excruciating social gatherings, but self-doubt is a virus that also infects every part of our lives—how we raise our kids, connect to our spouses and partners, do our work, and engage in the world. Thus, we learn to co-exist with it, chronically disappointed in failing to get with the program du jour. Low-grade self-loathing becomes part of our interior landscape, a noxious weed we whack at with affirmations and empowerment T-shirts, but never quite eradicate. We believe that one day, in the future, we will be our best self, but that day never arrives. Our lives become Groundhog Day, only instead of February 2 and Bill Murray, it's always the second week in January, when New Year's resolutions are in shambles and the self-hatred flows like the red wine you vowed to stop drinking, despite its antioxidant properties.

I swore off self-improvement on April 8, 2017. It was during a week when I was tracking every inhale and exhale with one of those fancy planners advertised to change your life. I have no clue why it was this particular bit of lunacy that led me to say fuck it all, but on the morning of April 8, moments after the alarm went off, I was already in a state. I'd read a thing about how you're supposed to awaken naturally. If you need to set an alarm, it was a sign you hadn't gotten enough sleep. Not getting enough sleep leads to elevated cortisol levels, which leads to a bunch of diseases *and* not being able to lose weight, and that day was the second day of my new whole clean-eating mindfulness challenge, which included awakening naturally, so I experienced the clear sense that I already wasn't doing it right. I hadn't actually *set* the alarm the night before. It was already set. On my phone. Which wasn't supposed to be on my bedside table in the first place, as dictated by some other digital detox protocol that I was also following half-heartedly.

It was 7:02 a.m. and I was angry at myself. I was aware of not feeling grateful—something else you're supposed to do upon waking—for living in a house with locking doors and a working furnace, plus the luxury of being able to do the whole clean-eating mindfulness challenge in the first place. Also, having a good man who loves me, snoring away next to me. I hadn't even gotten out of bed, and I was already depressed by my inadequacies, by the never-ending ambient noise in my head that I needed to do better. It was all so boring.

The whole point of what I was trying and failing to do was to live in a way that would make me happy, according to the current thinking on the need for fancy planners to improve your quality of life. But here's the thing: I'm *already* happy in the mornings. When I close my eyes at night, I'm a little excited by the thought of my first cup of coffee, dark roast with a splash of half-and-half, and a good game of Dead Hand with my dog, Rita.* The absurdity of laboring so mightily to achieve what I already had finally registered.

---

* To play Dead Hand: the first moment the dog noses your hand in the morning, you give her the best, deepest caress in your dog-petting arsenal. You scratch behind her ears, you rub her chest, you begin to pet her all the way down her back. Just when the dog closes her eyes in bliss, you "fall back asleep" and your hand goes dead. The dog waits for a moment, then starts nosing your hand a little, then, if she's Rita, flings it into the air. Then you burst out laughing, and start petting her again, just until her eyes close with bliss, etc., etc.

I decided to swear off self-improvement. Aside from the regular shoring up of the ruins that had become habit (dyeing my hair, a facial when I thought about it, steering clear of plaid), I was *done*. I was *quitting*. I was never going to get up earlier than I had to. I was never going to end my relationship with chips and guacamole. I was never going to be cool or hip or free from a certain degree of agita. I was never going to love card games or New Year's Eve. I was never going to stop taking online personality tests and then barking "what a load of crap!" out loud to the empty room or swear off astrology, which is also a load of crap, but I like thinking of myself as a Pisces Queen. I was never going to be a mysterious beauty. Serenity: not my bag. Neither is running a marathon (or a 10K, 5K, or any other "K"). I was done with programs, action plans, strategies, schemes, regimens, and ginormous planners that have you brainstorming the side dishes for Thanksgiving four years from now; I was always going to be a woman who embraced ideas that took her fancy with the slavering enthusiasm of a Labrador retriever, ate candy, lolled around reading a novel when she should be working, and had a bit of a muffin top.

My younger-man husband has long said that all he cared about, vis-à-vis the state of my naked bod, is that I'm "naked and smiling," and I've decided to take him at his word. I would make sure I ate my vegetables, did my walk/run around the neighborhood without my phone (and its library of podcasts) while admiring the beauty of nature, pet the dog, read books, and spent time with my daughter—now a young adult—and my friends. To lunging after the ever-receding mirage of the perfect me, I would say yeah, no, not happening.

This should be the part where I tell you how freeing it is to say fuck it all, but it wasn't that easy. I'd spent decades not feeling good enough and feeling guilty for not being able to do what I needed to do to improve myself. Before I could truly free myself, I had to confront the foundational emotion that fueled my need for never-ending self-improvement: shame.

The Voldemort of emotions, shame is so icky and intense no one wants to think about it, much less acknowledge it. In her early academic work, University of Houston research professor Brené Brown specialized exclusively on shame and its effect on women's lives. She tells a story in *I Thought It Was Just Me (But It Isn't)* about how when she would mention that her primary academic interest was shame, people wrinkled their noses, as if the toilet had backed up. Once, on a flight to give a talk, she struck up a conversation with her seatmate. Over the roar of the engine, the seatmate thought Brown said she was giving a speech on "women in chains." The seatmate was intrigued—how fascinating! When Brown said no, it's women *and shame*, the conversation abruptly ended, and the seatmate professed a sudden need to take a nap. People feel shame just *thinking* about all the things they feel ashamed about. I feel a little ashamed bringing shame up, especially when it's much more entertaining to riff on all the stupid stuff marketed to women that we can laugh at and roll our eyes about, then secretly google in the wee hours of a sleepless night.

Brown interviewed three hundred subjects over the course of six years, and the scope and depth of shame experienced by perfectly lovely women blew her mind. We feel the most shame around our appearance (90 percent of the women Brown spoke to felt shame about their bodies) and motherhood. Followed by: family, money and work, mental and physical health, sex, aging, religion, being stereotyped and labeled, and speaking out about and surviving trauma. The only thing women don't feel shame about, or so it appears, is the inability to throw a curveball or play "Bohemian Rhapsody" on the ukulele.

Shame, as Brown defines it, is ". . . the intensely painful feeling or experience of believing we are flawed and therefore unworthy of acceptance and belonging." That innocuous-seeming *therefore* connecting the two parts of the definition is a heartbreaker. Humans are hardwired to yearn to belong. Otherwise we wouldn't survive. Humans are also flawed, every one of us. We feel intense pain because we believe we are flawed—and we are—which leads to feeling *unworthy* of fulfilling the hardwired need to be accepted, to belong, and to be loved.

Shame is so noxious, most of us go to great lengths to try to develop coping mechanisms. We devote our lives to attempting to dig ourselves out of our shame prison with a teaspoon. Brown calls these behaviors shame screens. We move against our shame by becoming aggressive or trying to gain and maintain control over others; we move away from shame by with-drawing into ourselves and staying silent; we move toward our shame by doing what we can to gain approval. For competent, resourceful, can-do women, it's something of a Goldilocks situation. Aggression and domination is too hard; putting up and shutting up is too soft; but engaging in approval-seeking behavior is just right.

"Every day, in every way, I'm getting better and better," or so went the mantra Girl Scout Troop 203 recited at the end of each meeting, guided by our exuberant troop leader. Early twentieth-century French pharmacist and self-styled psychotherapist Émile Coué founded the Coué Method of "unconscious autosuggestion" based on this very mantra. It was popular in Europe and also, apparently, Whittier, California: long after I'd quit Girl Scouts and became a cheerleader in high school, we closed every practice with this affirmation. Every day, in every way, I'm getting better and better.

The pot of gold at the end of every self-improvement program is a sense of accomplishment (at the end of the day the most important pat on the back is the one you give yourself) and happiness, comprised of gaining approval and a sense of belonging, knowing that you're one step closer to being a perfect, unimpeachable female according to the demands of the times. The always-improving female is doing the correct work of her gender. She is tending to her knitting and staying in her lane. She is cheerful, selfless, accommodating, and smoking hot, regardless of whether the sociological trend du jour has her attachment parenting at home or taking a pink sledgehammer to the glass ceiling in the office, or a combo of both. And she is doing it all effortlessly, or so she works to make it appear, because to seem too focused on ourselves is selfish, and thus unacceptable.

It's an elegant trap, fashioned by a consumeristic society that benefits from keeping women in shame and obsessed with self-improvement. We are taught to believe that if we can just improve ourselves, we can escape the terrible, shame-induced feelings of humiliation and alienation. It's shame that drives us to seek self-improvement, but shame is also the result when we fail to attain the impossible goal that is supposed to free us from the shame that drove us to seek the improvement in the first place.

Shame is so potent, in part because it operates on many levels, sometimes all at once. As children, the scolding we receive from our parents or caregivers is often internalized as shame. As we move into the world, peers and teachers join the chorus. We feel shame when we get our periods and, depending on the culture in which we're raised, spend our lives ashamed of occupying a female body.

The experience of shame generally involves another voice in our head, whether it's one we've manufactured in the form of self-admonishment (we've let ourselves down again—by eating the chocolate cake on day five of the diet, by relapsing, by being too weak or lazy to stick to whatever plan we set on Monday) or literally one we've heard in the past or present telling us we're not good enough (our mother, our teacher, our boss, our partner). It's always a voice/an "other" that we permit to pass judgment on us, causing us to feel shame.

This internal chatter accompanies us as we move through our days, encountering situations that cause us shame in the here and now. But here is where we have a chance to lighten our shame load a bit, and when it comes to reducing our sense of shame, every little bit helps.

During Brown's investigation, when she asked her subjects what sorts of experiences caused their sense of shame to spike, she noticed that many women began their sentences with "I don't want people to see me as . . ." or "I don't want to be seen as . . ."

We lose weight for our health and to feel good, but also so people don't think we're fat. (More than mere vanity, during the last decade weight discrimination against women in the workplace has increased by 66 percent.) We work out with the rigor of an Olympic gymnast for sleeveless dress season, so people won't make jokes about bat wings behind our backs. We spend a fortune at the hair stylist every six weeks so that people will think we are younger. We volunteer for a pointless task at work so that people will think we're a team player. We exhaust ourselves throwing the best birthday parties for our kids, aware of what other moms might be saying. We fret over whether our children are fitting in, and what we can do to help *them* avoid being harshly judged. On and on it goes. Perhaps it would be worth the tedium of living a life in which we felt like our own jailers if it achieved what we hoped, if it freed us from the shame of being judged. But it doesn't, and it never will, and not for the reasons we might expect.

If you're engaged in a version of the above for the validation you seek from others, you can quit now. It turns out, no one is thinking about you. No one is seeing you in a way you don't want to be seen, because everyone is thinking about themselves and how *they* want to be seen. If we're all hardwired to seek acceptance and belonging, the person you're worried about judging you is also worried about how you are judging them.

A groundbreaking piece of research published in 2018 by neurologists Meghan L. Meyer and Matthew D. Lieberman suggests the reason we tend to always think about ourselves. By studying the activity of the medial prefrontal cortex, they determined that the part of our brain responsible for self-reflection kicks into gear whenever our attention is not captured by an external demand. If, for example, you're driving down the street and you suddenly need to brake to avoid hitting a pedestrian, in the split second when you realize you need to put your foot on the brake, you are not thinking about yourself. But every moment leading up to that reaction, and every moment leading from it, your brain is occupied with a variety of thoughts about yourself.

The part of our brain governing automatic self-absorption is a vast and complex neurological web called the default mode network. The DMN processes our memories, creates and stores our self-perception, and evaluates our emotional state and the emotional states of others. In 1929, Hans Berger, inventor of the electroencephalogram, posited that our brains are always active, but it wasn't until the development of the PET (positron-emission tomography) scan and the fMRI in the 1990s that neuroscientists were able to observe the DMN in action. The growing sophistication of technology, including computational analyses, has given rise to an explosion of interest in the DMN, the place where, according to Jessica R. Andrews-Hanna, writing in the *Neuroscientist*, our "highly personally significant and goal-directed thoughts" about our past and our future reside.

This is reassuring news for several reasons. First, because it means we're hardwired for a certain amount of selfishness; we shouldn't feel guilty about thinking about ourselves, because it's literally our default mode. Second, and more pertinent to this discussion, most of the time when we're feeling judged by others, *we are judging ourselves in a way we imagine someone else might judge us.*

When my daughter, Fiona, was in eighth grade, she came home weeping one day. A girl she'd thought was a friend told her best friend that my daughter was a "low-key slut." I had no idea what that was, but it couldn't be good. After I made a batch of blueberry bread, my girl's favorite comfort snack, and hugged her and indulged in a fantasy of finding and strangling that so-called friend, I consoled Fiona by telling her that it wasn't about her, but about the friend. Sure enough, when Fiona's best friend confronted the girl spreading the gossip, she admitted that she was jealous of Fiona and her popularity.

Fiona was relieved, and I was relieved to have been able to offer some parental wisdom that wasn't the usual platitude.

The moment we accept that people aren't judging us, but rather judging themselves and projecting their own dissatisfaction with themselves onto us, is the moment we begin to liberate ourselves from the bonds of self-improvement. But it's not easy. As you'll see, a lot of people have a lot invested in keeping women in shame and focused on chasing the fantasy of perfection. But we can fight those forces. Instead of trying to escape the shame of being imperfect by resorting to trying to "fix" ourselves, let's take some time to see how we got here. Let's have today be the day we begin imagining life as the "come as you are" party it should be.

CHAPTER 2

The Great Female Self-Improvement Bamboozlement

To free us from the expectations of others, to give us back to ourselves—there lies the great, the singular power of self-respect.
—Joan Didion, "Self-Respect: Its Source, Its Power"

Before I swore off self-improvement I would look at my phone over my morning coffee. All the productivity gurus said this was a terrible habit, but I did it anyway, something I already felt bad about. After a few minutes of scrolling, I was reminded of all the ways I didn't measure up. I hadn't spoken to another human being yet, hadn't even read an email. I'm pretty sure no one was judging me or seeing me in any specific way—in part because anyone who might have been was also looking at *their* phone. Instead, I was starting my day with the messages of a hundred ads thrumming in my head. My parents or family weren't shaming me, nor were my friends, coworkers, or anyone in my social sphere. No human was involved in the making of my despair and self-loathing.

The most successful way to sell something to a woman has always been to bamboozle her. Convincingly create an imaginary problem—ideally something she's never thought about so as to induce complete panic—then save the day by providing just the right product to set her mind at ease. Ads targeted at women are designed to stir up emotions and have been since the dawn of advertising. With relative ease, we can be manipulated into doubting ourselves. We care less about the price or function of something and more about fixing what we've been told was wrong with us, and it's been this way for a hundred years. No one alive in today's modern world has escaped its influence.

Behold an advertisement in a 1919 issue of *Ladies' Home Journal* for a deodorant called Odorono: "Within the Curve of a Woman's Arm, a frank discussion of a subject too often avoided."[*] The accompanying illustration shows a handsome couple in evening wear. He is considerably taller than she. Her slender arm is raised. Her delicate hand rests upon his manly shoulder. They appear to be waltzing, but in fact she's got him backed into the corner of a balcony, where he's obviously trying escape her

---

[*] Within this sentence some shitty grammatical syntax as well.

eye-watering BO. The mailbag at *LHJ* burst with outraged letters. Alluding to the way women smell was scandalous, tasteless to the point of immorality. But sales of Odorono shot through the roof.

The smell of our breath could also ruin our lives. In 1923 the makers of Listerine mouthwash worried we would be "often a bridesmaid, but never a bride." A 1923 ad campaign featured Edna, who "like every woman, her primary ambition was to marry." But "as her birthdays crept gradually toward that tragic thirty mark, marriage seemed farther from her life than ever." But Edna's story ends happily. Her problem was merely halitosis, nothing a slug of Listerine couldn't fix. This ad campaign increased Listerine's profits by 4000 percent in six years and has become a legend of advertising history.

Men haven't escaped the manipulations of the marketing and advertising industry, but women are the titans of shopping, responsible for more than three-quarters of all consumer spending. Because we drive the entire economy with our handbag and shapewear purchases, our gym memberships, weekly salon appointments, and, not incidentally, the tons of stuff we buy to keep the household afloat, food on the table, and the kids in monstrously expensive sneakers, the advertising industry spends its billions focused on selling primarily to us. There's no marketing deep state (or none that my research turned up, anyway) that uses targeted advertising to control women, to keep them mired in self-loathing and focused on what they can purchase to improve themselves, but that's more or less the result.

In 2018 women spent forty trillion dollars worldwide on consumer goods, up from twenty-seven trillion in 2013. A 2019 study showed that 94 percent of females between the ages of fifteen and thirty-five spend over an hour a day shopping online. A 2015 article in *Forbes* called "Top 10 Things Everyone Should Know About Women Consumers" begins with "If the consumer economy had a sex, it would be female." The post advises ". . . study[ing] women as you would a foreign market." The *Today* show reported a study showing that with the money a woman spends on cosmetics over the course of a lifetime, she could afford to buy a house.

My intention in trotting out these statistics is not to whip up shame around shopping. As cultural critic Ellen Willis pointed out in a 1970 essay on women and consumerism, the primacy of the marketplace, and the socializing and relationship building that takes place there, is an ancient and communal human activity. Women purchased food and household goods to take care of their families. They bartered, managed their budgets, and procured all the stuff necessary for domestic life. Only at the rise of the twentieth century did the notion of shopping as a leisure time activity take hold, perpetuated and driven by advertising. It made women feel as if they were in control of their own lives, and to a degree, this was not untrue. My housewife mom prided herself on tracking down sales and finding the best deal. That most of the time it was for stuff we didn't need only reaffirms the manipulative power of advertising.

You could google old-time ads all day long for a cheap laugh, but the joke is on us. These silly ads with their alarming taglines and melodramatic stories were educating us, training us in the consumeristic two-step: identify with the woman being shamed in the advertisement, who then "cures" her inferiority complex by purchasing the product.

Between World War I and II, Madison Avenue found itself stymied. Smoking had become a huge pastime. It was glamorous and seductive, and every movie star did it. The problem: despite the many brands, cigarettes looked alike and smoked alike. They were all pretty much the same cigarettes. Why choose Camel when Lucky Strike would do? Cigarettes were also a product no one needed, except smokers, who, at the time, were unaware that nicotine was addictive.

Enter the clever tactic of selling a lifestyle the consumer would come to associate with the product. Marlboro was originally called Marlborough, named for the street where cigarette maker Philip Morris operated his factory, and was targeted as a smoke for women, with its "ladylike filter." It was no different from any other filtered cigarette, and its sales were modest. Then, in 1950, after the release of a major British study linking smoking to cancer, Philip Morris began advertising the filter as a disease preventative. Marlborough became Marlboro and rebranded as a cigarette for a man's man who was smart enough to be concerned about his health. The image of the rugged, handsome, independent Marlboro Man who "came to the flavor" was born and inspires would-be cowboys to this day.[*]

Philip Morris also manufactured Virginia Slims, and in 1973 launched a campaign that harnessed the prevailing winds of second-wave feminism. The ads featured "liberated" slim, pretty, glamorous young women rocking the latest fashion, who personified the tagline, "You've come a long way, baby." Sepia-toned photographs appeared in the upper corner or on the side of the image of the comely smoker, illustrating how far "baby" had come. One showed a woman churning butter beside a parody of the lyrics of "I Want a Girl (Just Like the Girl That Married Dear Old Dad)": *She'll wash the floors | Polish up the doors | And never make me mad | She won't smoke | Or be a suffragette | She will always be my loving pet . . .*

The campaign caused a stir: feminists were disgruntled at the use of the word *baby*, while traditionalists decried the celebration of "women libbers." Teenage girls, in the meantime, felt as if smoking Virginia Slims empowered them to tear up the world. In their hot pants and suede boots, birth control pills and ciggies tucked in their shoulder bags, they would be in-charge women so different from their mothers![†]

But what had really come a long way was advertising. By the

---

[*] Not to mention male porn stars, gay and straight alike.

[†] That this blockbuster ad campaign also inspired young women to blacken their young pink lungs with tar and nicotine was something no one seemed to care about.

mid-twentieth century, consumers would no longer require a hokey, hypothetical narrative to connect the dots.

Synecdoche is a literary device in which a part stands in for the whole. On TV, a close-up of a woman handing over her credit card to someone else signifies a purchase. We don't have to see her flipping through racks of clothes, trying them on, then deciding on this or that. We've been trained by a lifetime of TV and movie consumption to know what handing over the plastic means. Our comprehension is sophisticated. The hand itself also communicates information. Is it soft and plump with polished nails and golden rings? Is it grubby, with nails bitten to the quick? What does this tell us about the owner of the card? We don't need to see her in relation to another human being. We don't need a story to convey the message, however subtly, that something is wrong with us, and it needs to be fixed.

A study published in the *Journal of Consumer Research* in 2011 revealed that just a photograph of a beauty product—a bottle of perfume, a stylish stiletto, a tube of lipstick—made female subjects feel worse about themselves. There was no attendant copy, not a word. Just an image that evokes what we've all come to think of as a successful (i.e., beautiful) woman is enough to make us feel as if we are lacking. The researchers learned something else: the distress their subjects felt did not lead to "lower buying intentions," but just the opposite. We buy more when we feel bad about ourselves, and we feel bad about ourselves a lot.

By the age of thirteen I'd gotten the message that part of being female was never believing you were good enough. I was going through a mad phase of creating large collages on poster board using pictures torn from magazines. I remember an ad for the Little Fibber Bra, featuring a large pear with the message, "This is no shape for a girl." Also, a diet soda ad showing a slender and smoking-hot young woman in a red bikini trying to button her jeans. "You can do it. Pepsi can help." My mind was completely blown by the pervy 1974 ads for Love's Baby Soft body spray, featuring pouty-lipped teen sexpots in white puffed-sleeved dresses cuddling teddy bears and the tagline, "Because innocence is sexier than you think."

Repurposing the images from the ads into devastatingly cool collages did nothing to dilute the message: a girl could not hope to feel accepted, loved, and safe unless she was beautiful, and to be beautiful was complicated, if not impossible. Since everything about our bodies could be improved, it meant that every part was unacceptable unless it *was* improved. A girl's less-than-perfect breasts could be fixed by buying a Playtex padded bra. A girl's not-white-enough, not-bright-enough teeth could be fixed by brushing with Pepsodent. A girl's plethora of hair problems (not enough body, not enough shine, not enough volume, horrifying, social life–destroying frizz) could be fixed by a myriad of hair products.

Those early messages of inadequacy, gleaned from the ads in *Seventeen*, gathered into a steady stream of lowish self-esteem that flowed beneath my life, regardless of whether I succeeded or failed, was loved or lost. It's a mark of advertising's eternal might that even as I grew up and went to college and suffered the early death of my mother, got married and had a child, then divorced, got married again and acquired two stepchildren, then divorced again, then married again, built a rickety career as an author, traveled all over the world, read and wrote, bought and sold homes, adored and said goodbye to several great dogs, and recently moved from Portland, Oregon, to a tiny village in the south of France, I've never been able to deny what advertising was selling, which is a fundamental sense of inadequacy. No experience matters, no maturity matters, no knowledge that I'm being manipulated. My feelings are stirred up in a way they've been designed to, and those feelings make me wonder if maybe the ad is right.

At the airport recently I flipped through a copy of a glossy women's magazine. Airports are the last places in America that have well-stocked magazine racks, presumably because there are still people who view a plane ride as a chance to unplug. I spied an ad for a $4000 purse, a lion-colored calfskin leather shoulder bag with a gold clasp. It was photographed in a manner that evoked style, class, affluence, and sexiness. Even though I knew exactly what was going on, that extremely well-paid professionals designed and created this image to stir up inchoate yearning, I felt a pinch of despair: *I am not the kind of sophisticated woman who carries a bag like that, nor could I afford it even if I was. Nor would I buy it even if I could afford it, because is there anything more vulgar than a $4000* *handbag?* . . . Around and around my thoughts went. My intellect was of no use to me, even though I knew from experience that women's magazines basically exist to pour gasoline on the fire of our obsession with self-improvement.

One day a dozen years ago or so, an editor from *Self* emailed, asking if I would contribute my best weight-loss tip to a feature on no bullshit dieting.* I wrote back to say I would be happy to do this, as I was in possession of the only tip that anyone would ever need: "Eat less, move more." She didn't write back. After a few days, I wrote to her again. She answered quickly, "So sorry, but our readers are interested in diets that are more science-based, possibly including some good supplements."

I knew how women's magazines aided and abetted our quest for perfection, but I was still naïve enough to believe that a "no bullshit dieting" feature would not push the same old complicated eating plans that consumed a woman's every waking moment. The no bullshit dieting feature was bullshit, and I realized in that moment the female compulsion for self-improvement would be exploited until the last woman alive was still fretting about her thigh gap while running for her life during the zombie apocalypse.

Even when you're minding your own business reading a serious newspaper about serious world events, there's no escaping advertising. There I am one Sunday morning, reading the *New*

---

* This was in a time before *tips* had been rebranded as the sexier-sounding *hacks.*

York Times. I flip through the *Style* magazine, past all the ads for things only the 1 percent can afford, thinking maybe there are some cool clothes. My grandmother was a couturiere, and I learned to sew about the time I learned to read, so I love to see what's up in the world of outrageous, arty, completely unaffordable fashion.

I come upon a headline: "How You Can Get Glowing Skin with Minimal Makeup." Who is the readership for this article, which is just an advertisement dressed up in editorial clothing? Women who prefer their skin to possess "a subtle dewiness that suggests the afterglow of a hike or yoga session." Hell, yeah! Before this moment, I didn't fully comprehend that there was an appropriate degree of skin dewiness that I should strive to obtain, but it makes sense. On one end of the spectrum there's hot flash during a heatwave, on the other, dried apple head doll. Now that I know, I cannot unknow.

The solution lies in following this five-step routine: daily exfoliation ($195) followed by weekly microblading ($150) to make sure you start with a smooth, light-reflecting surface; replace old foundation with one of the new water-based tinted gels ($65); massage area around eye with an ice cube to reduce puffiness and tighten skin before applying concealer ($65) with a special sponge-tip applicator; pat on special highlighter that "combines antioxidant-rich jojoba oil with a peachy-brown tint" ($75); follow with a spritz of extra dew-creating hydrating mist ($45).

I am a complete sucker for skin care products. I want all of this, even the unpleasantly futuristic microblading thing. If I had $595 to spare, I would go online and order up all this shit right now. But I don't have $595 to spare, and that makes me feel bad about myself, my career, my ability to manage money, and my skin, which is smooth but neither glowing nor dewy. Really, the only thing that made me feel marginally better about falling for articles like this one again and again was that Simone de Beauvoir wasn't immune to this sort of thing either. She may have said, "Society cares for the individual only so far as he is profitable." But she also said, "Buying is a profound pleasure." So, there you go.

Before the digital age we were exposed to advertising through much slower forms of media. TV and radio commercials could be ridiculously memorable, but radios and televisions could be turned off.* They didn't come with you everywhere you went. Glossy magazines sat in a row on the newsstands, minding their own business. Maybe you had a magazine subscription or two. They were powerful message bearers, but after they arrived, you flipped through them, sniffed the perfume ads, then dropped them on the coffee table or decorative basket beside the commode. Or they became fodder for adolescent art projects.

---

* I wish I were an Oscar Mayer Wiener / that is what I'd truly like to be / 'cause if I were an Oscar Mayer Wiener / everyone would be in love with me.

These leisurely delivery systems allowed us to forget for long stretches of time that we and our lives were imperfect and in need of fixing. Our self-esteem may have plunged upon reading that full-page ad for boots worn by a tan supermodel in a gold bikini, but we couldn't stare at that picture indefinitely—well, maybe you could if you were stoned out of your mind—and then real life intervened and distracted us from our feelings of inadequacy. We had things to do that helped us reassert our self-image as a human being with agency. The homely demands of reality saved us. The passage of time, during which we lived our lives, free from the onslaught of advertisements, provided a bit of a corrective. Back then, reality could still compete with the emotions of yearning and self-abasement churned up by advertising. We were not being waterboarded nonstop with the message that we needed to improve ourselves.

Social media may not be the fount of all evil, but it's also naïve to assume it's simply the next iteration of a glossy women's magazine. A seductive digital mind shaper, these platforms condition us moment by moment to long for other lives, always better than our own. No matter how lousy our habitual scrolling makes us feel—and there is now plenty of evidence that social media makes us more anxious, depressed, and despairing—we still don't unfollow someone who makes us feel fat, ugly, poor, or unloved. We become *more* attached; we don't just "follow" them, we *follow* them. Our inner thirteen-year-old is rekindled. Oh, to be like the popular girl! To have that hair, husband, kids, stamina, "passion," slender fingers on which to display delicate gold rings, that perfect recipe for a refreshing healthy pasta salad, that evolved spiritual outlook, that collection of equally cool friends with whom to raise fish bowl–size goblets of wine.

While social scientists and psychologists are dutifully performing carefully designed longitudinal studies to assess whether our heavy phone usage is destroying what's left of our attention spans, rewiring our brains, and making us itchy with impatience when forced to endure a face-to-face encounter, advertisers have quickly figured out how to leverage our addiction.

As I write this, the average cell phone user picks up her device fifty-two times a day. Allowing for eight hours of sleep, this works out to about every twenty minutes, or three times an hour. Three times an hour, day in day out, we're assaulted with messages and advertisements, and they aren't just any old messages and ads. Thanks to the wonder of the algorithm, they have been fine-tuned to stir up our deepest insecurities. Doing the math, that means eighty times a day we get a message, however brief, of who we aren't, what we don't have, and what we are never likely to have unless we take proper measures. Unless we do something to improve ourselves.

Just now I checked my bank balance. I logged out of my bank app and opened Instagram. The first sponsored ad to pop up before I began my customary slack-jawed scroll featured a tall woman of a certain age. She was still catwalk slim, with immaculate posture. She strode into frame wearing a brightly colored caftan that looked like something Eileen Fisher might design for South Sea royalty. But the ad wasn't about the caftan; it was about a webinar for women and money. "A year to get rich with purpose. This is how you transform your financial world."

Nothing makes me break out in a cold sweat more than the suggestion that I need to get my financial act together. I felt terrible about myself, immediately. Terrible that I couldn't rock a brightly colored caftan in any way that didn't make me look like your crazy aunt gone to seed, terrible that I wasn't thinner, and terrible that I have the money-managing skills of a seven-year-old whose primary source of income is the tooth fairy. I am not a webinar person—really, isn't it just someone blathering at you on Zoom?—but I was tempted to click on this one.

For the next three minutes I continued to scroll, during which the almighty algorithm presented me with sponsored ads for:

Cute suede ankle boots

Salad with homegrown greens

Ultracomfort bra

Yoga philosophy reading list

Gorgeous black-and-white photograph of a woman washing her thick black hair

"The Wellness Special"

Recipe for baking a gluten-free, dairy-free chocolate cake

Picture of a bunch of women with tiny asses celebrating #globalrunningday

A celebrity wearing super cute $185 shoes made of recycled something or other

Customize your very own bangle stack!

Facetune app 2

This anti-aging cream really works

Beautiful tiny cabin

Have you tried our bestselling tinted lip sculpting oil?

Sleep like a baby

Perfecting skin tint. Sheer, beautiful coverage. Breathable formula autofits to skin

Radical creative productivity

Lean legs and thighs in 14 days

Install this app and get your personal fasting plan

Heist: revolutionary summer shapewear has arrived

Taking your writing business to the next level

You are everything you think

I don't imagine this list makes you feel as despondent as it does me. This specific assortment of come-ons was designed to make *me* feel crappy. You have your *own* list, derived from your own clicks and likes. Although we prefer not to think about it, it pays to recall that the free social media platforms to which we've attached ourselves like a barnacle to the hull of a ship are designed to do one thing: hoover up our data, then blast us with personally targeted ads that feed into our concerns, worries, obsessions, and desires.

It gets more complicated. Flowing alongside sponsored ads is a gushing stream of chipper posts created by so-called influencers, all peddling a similar version of the elusive feminine ideal. Will Storr, writing in *Selfie: How We Became So Self-*

Obsessed and What It's Doing to Us, pretty much nails it. "It's not difficult to detect the general model of ideal selfhood that the culture of today has come up with. It's usually depicted as an extroverted, slim, beautiful, individualistic, optimistic, hardworking, socially aware yet high-self-esteeming global citizen with entrepreneurial guile and a selfie camera."

Influencers were the beginning of the end of self-improvery for me. Sponsored ads never got to me: they were labeled and obvious. The cloying, inspirational messages from the stratospherically famous were also relatively easy to enjoy, without my feeling as if I needed to drop everything and do a juice fast or get myself a productivity guru. But beyond the ads and beneath the famous, a peppy army of pretty, photogenic, articulate women endlessly shilled products and programs they promised would improve us and our lives, and I didn't know what to make of them. The influencers I followed were enough like me to give me a glimpse of what my life would be like if I just buckled down and improved myself. The very fact of their existence, adorably gardening, enjoying a communal meal outdoors at a big wooden table with a bouquet of sunflowers stuck in a chipped jug, snuggling with their dogs as they read a popular yet enriching novel 'neath an alpaca throw, flung me into a panic. If they could have this life, couldn't I? Or more to the point, shouldn't I?

Before the turn of the twenty-first century the division between the image makers and the image consumers was still clear. No matter how many thousands of advertisements and photoshopped fashion spreads we consumed, we knew they came from people who were paid to make them. Selling us stuff was just their job, the same way defense attorneys make a living ensuring the rights of psycho killers and scumbags are protected. It took me a while to realize it was the same with influencers, with their faux affection for their followers (many of whom have turned out to be fake) and their contracts to mention a product a specific number of times. It was their job, and part of their job was to make it not look like advertising.*

There's a subset of influencers I've had some experience with in real life: successful cisgender heteronormative middle-class white women (like me) who've managed to make a great success of their lives. They practice something Canadian writer and feminist marketing consultant Kelly Diels identified as FLEB, Female Lifestyle Empowerment Brand. FLEB is a marketing narrative driven largely by female entrepreneurs, most of whom were at one time in the "display professions"— actresses, musicians, or models. On their Instagram feeds the FLEB entrepreneurs come across as best girlfriends, generously offering their life lessons, exercise tips, and skin care

---

* Since I began writing this book the tide seems to have turned against influencers. Too many seem to have been caught purchasing fake followers and retweets, and advertisers began to get suspicious when their most followed influencer was only able to sell fourteen tubs of detoxing protein powder.

secrets. The underlying message is "I'm the best, most improved version of myself, and you can be too." Predictably, the result is not empowerment but, rather, says Diels, to encourage other women to "be hotter, tauter, richer, more positive, more productive, and more serene. In other words, be more of what our mainstream media and culture already demands of women."

It's the same old bamboozlement, reconfigured for the digital age.

The jewel in the FLEB crown is goop, Gwyneth Paltrow's lifestyle and e-commerce site. Founded a thousand years ago in internet time, the site still claims two million wellness seekers per month. There they purchase $185 "active" botanical serum and hoover up pseudo-scientific medical advice. The most famous, for which Paltrow was fined $145,000 (pocket change) for unsubstantiated claims, involved Jade Eggs for Your Yoni, inserted to "balance hormones, regulate menstrual cycles, prevent uterine prolapse, and increase bladder control." Vox reported in 2018 that despite the ruling, goop was still selling the infamous eggs, with a revised promise that using them would "increase sexual energy and pleasure." In the summer of 2019, the Jade Egg was still available, minus the description of what it does or why you would want one. What remains is a wonderfully surreal bit of genuinely useful information: eggs are pre-drilled for a string add-on; unwaxed dental floss is recommended.

Every dustup in the press about goop's dubious claims does nothing to discredit the operation.* Her followers still click on "What I Packed for My Weekend at Shou Sugi Ban House, a Gorgeous New Hamptons Spa," which features a $35 packet of "The Martini" Emotional Detox Bath Soak.

It's easy to poke fun at Paltrow, who is, after all, just an attractive, very clean-looking businesswoman/snake oil salesperson and, at one time, a pretty good actor. It's hardly her fault that we're happy to abandon all reason in the hope of becoming a fully detoxed spirit warrior. Of course, the other thing she's selling is class identity. The invisible, and bogus, free gift that comes with a $125 tub of exfoliator is the illusion that we are in Paltrow's tax bracket and can easily afford the shockingly overpriced stuff she sells.

Over the years, I've been contracted to ghostwrite books for a handful of prominent FLEB entrepreneurs. Each one was a powerhouse in her own right. Each one rose to success in her field under her own steam. Each one has stamina, grit, smarts, and ambition. Each one has struggled and triumphed. I was awed and inspired by all of them. They are also rich women in a rich nation, which makes all the difference in how they

---

* Bashing goop has become a small but mighty subgenre of digital culture reporting. Some of the pieces are so laugh-your-ass-off hilarious that reading them has got to be good for your health. *New York* magazine's The Cut opened a story about the supposed benefits of coffee enemas with "Have you ever looked at a freshly brewed pot of coffee and thought, 'That should go in my butt'? No? Well, according to goop, you're missing out."

live. While they are devoted to authenticity, these women were shy and unforthcoming when it came to addressing the freedom that goes with having boatloads of money. They could not very well admit that their (well-earned) wealth allows them the freedom to invest, literally, in "radical" self-care, wellness, spirituality, satisfying their curiosities and yearnings through travel, and pursuing their passions and goals. For all the talk about transparency, it's the one thing they are not comfortable talking about, and the thing that makes all the difference.

I know, because every time I brought up money during our work sessions it would be the beginning of the end of our partnerships. I would never say anything as crass as "but you're a millionaire—no wonder you can go to India for six months, even if you did sleep on the floor at the ashram." I would try to broach the subject diplomatically. "Um, shouldn't we reassure the reader that your ideas are useful to everyone, even the mom with three kids, two jobs, and a neighbor with insomnia and a drum kit, who is looking for a way to incorporate meditation into her life?"

As I said, these were very smart women. In their defense, few of us have been raised to discuss money openly and honestly. They probably saw and see themselves as average wage earners, and certainly they didn't want to come off as being *privileged*, a member of the 1 percent in good standing. They could see that I had issues with the parts of their well-meaning philosophies that could only be given so much attention because they had the time and the money and the privilege to do so. One had an entire walk-in closet devoted to her purse collection. One had a $900 French candle on the table in her entryway. When their assistants brought in healthy food—well, say no more. They *had* assistants.

I have a not-unsuccessful writing career, but I have never had an assistant to bring in healthy food, unless you count my husband bringing me the occasional cranberry juice and grilled cheese. I want to make this clear: I don't begrudge them their purse collections, their high-three-figure candles, their assistants and helpers and trainers and private chefs and personal tattoo artists. I liked these women. Even after I was fired by some of them, I liked them. I still like them. What I disagree with is their underlying message: that with the proper thinking, essential oils, and plenty of greens you too can have a life like theirs. It's nonsense. The biggest real problem most of us have is how to pay the bills. How to pay our taxes. How to afford our medication. How to pay for a new water heater or braces for the kids (and even that problem is one of affluence). How to carve out a half hour a day where something is not required of us. Most of what they're peddling does nothing to help solve the challenge of making ends meet.

Carina Chocano, author of *You Play the Girl: On Playboy Bunnies, Stepford Wives, Train Wrecks & Other Mixed Messages*, wrote an article in the August 2019 issue of *Vanity Fair* chronicling the rise of some lesser-known practitioners of FLEB—the Instagram micro-influencers of Byron Bay, Australia. A beach town on the northeastern coast of New South Wales, Byron

Bay was once a hippie enclave, but is now the dead cool hub of "midtier family lifestyle micro-influencers," including a troupe of attractive "murfers" (mom surfers) who are practitioners of "slow" living, raising their equally beautiful children with wooden toys, no screens, impromptu picnics, "surf seshes," and cheerful hipster husbands who go along for the ride.

The piece begins: "Courtney Adamo's minimalist, Shaker-style kitchen is gorgeous, but you already know that if you follow her. . . . With its clapboard cupboards, wooden stools, bulk dry goods in mason jars, Blanc Marble countertops ('slightly more expensive than the Carrara,' she explains in a blog post about her kitchen renovation, 'but we are so happy with the decision'), Dunlin Chelsea Pendant Lights ($669 each), SMEG refrigerator ($2,870), Lacanche oven and stove ('range cooker of my dreams' and, at about $10,000, a 'splurge'), the kitchen is like a scene out of Little House on the Trust Fund Prairie. (@courtneyadamo, 250K Instagram followers)."

In her piece, Chocano worked hard to differentiate the five women from one another, but the first paragraph is so good, and so damning, few could see past Adamo's $10,000 "range cooker of my dreams." Chocano's Twitter feed documents the confused response. Some followers thought the piece was "delicious," and named their favorite murfer, others loved the takedown of these women and their disingenuous promotion of privilege, and others wagged their fingers at Chocano's apparent criticism of other women.

There's something futuristic and *Black Mirror*-ish about

transforming your life into an aestheticized performance to sell products. It's one thing to enslave yourself to creating a false narrative that spotlights products you are being paid to plug as part of your "brand," and another thing entirely to monetize and exploit your family life.

On the other hand, I was deeply covetous of those fucking $669 pendant lights. It's safe to say I've never had a single thought about pendant lights before reading about Adamo's. I don't think I was clear on how a pendant light differed from, like, a hanging lamp. Thus, in thirty seconds I'd become the poster girl for mimetic desire.

Mimetic desire is the psychological mechanism that makes influencers influential. One of our basic human impulses is to want what people we think are cool want. They have it, we want it, and together that escalates the value of the object. Look no further than the trend among the moms of Brooklyn's Park Slope to wear clogs and affix a brightly colored hand-woven Salt strap onto their Fendi handbag. These straps could have come straight from the guitar of the smelliest, most tone-deaf hippie in Haight-Ashbury—really, they're no different—but because the cool moms have them, those who perceive themselves as less cool also want them. Thus, my position vis-à-vis the fucking $669 pendant lights.

Pioneered by twentieth-century French philosopher and lit-erary scholar René Girard, mimetic desire is more than mere imitation of behavior or acquisition; you find yourself *want-ing* the same thing your role model wants. In the case of so many influencers, as it is with goop, it's a level of affluence most of us can never hope to achieve. Unless—or so we tell ourselves—we click on the link, join the program, go to the seminar, purchase the product. It raises our hopes before it dashes them. Once again, we feel the pinch of self-loathing that eventually sends us straight into the arms of another self-improvement regime. We've spent our time, energy, attention, and hard-earned cash, and have nothing but bad feelings about ourselves to show for it.

But there's good, very practical news.

You really can wean yourself off compulsive phone checking. Make some rules for yourself—not too many, or it will start seeming like self-improvery. Figure out ways to make it inconvenient to pick up your phone. Fling it to the bottom of your purse so it's a hassle to dig it out in public. Remove all but the essential apps. Vow to check social media only on your laptop and give yourself a time limit. On Instagram hide every sponsored ad that makes you feel even a wee bit lousy. (I always also report the ad as being inappropriate, just for kicks.) I'm not suggesting that you delete your social media accounts or trade in your smartphone for a flip phone. We're too far down the digital road for that. But the fewer times you pick up your phone, the fewer times the fire hose of advertising blasts you with messages that make you doubt yourself, the less power it will have over you. The less power modern consumer culture has over you, the greater your chances of becoming reacquainted with and reclaiming your True Self.

CHAPTER 3

It's Complicated: Self-Improvement for Girls

To be feminine is to show oneself as weak, futile, passive, and docile. The girl is supposed not only to primp and dress herself up but also to repress her spontaneity and substitute for it the grace and charm she has been taught by her elder sisters. Any self-assertion will take away from her femininity and her seductiveness.

—Simone de Beauvoir, *The Second Sex*

I didn't give a thought to self-improvement until seventh grade. Before that I wanted to *do* stuff better. Surf, ride a unicycle, walk on my hands, draw a box in perfect perspective, hone my jump shot, make a bomb using a Strike Anywhere match and a tennis ball. But once I'd acquired breasts and a box of Kotex in the cupboard beneath the bathroom sink, I was informed by my mother, and mass culture, that *looking* better should be my goal. My mother's primary concern became my height, weight, complexion, furry eyebrows, and "thunder thighs," all of which conveyed to me that whatever basic human strengths I might possess, feminine charm was not one of them.

Oh, how I longed to portray myself as some preternaturally self-possessed teen who knew her self-worth and thought her mother was a sad relic, pushing her sad outdated ideas. But I was cursed with a pragmatic nature. My mother was totally right. In the small world of my Southern California public high school, it was plain to see that the boys I liked preferred girls who were pretty and deliciously docile, with their long eyelashes, silky hair, and bewitching impassivity. And anyway, by then my veins were thrumming with estrogen, and I was happy to bid adieu to the snarly haired, cuticle-chewing, too-short, pants-wearing tomboy galumphing around the neighborhood.

A witty feminist quote about the tyranny of being born female and the pressure to conform to codified standards of beauty would fit in nicely right about here, but it's a cliché. Regardless of how many waves of feminism roll through, for women, beauty was and is the coin of the realm. Yesterday I asked my stepdaughter how *her* stepdaughter was managing middle school. She laughed and shrugged. "She's having a great time. She's thin and blond."

The summer between seventh and eighth grade I figured out how to iron my hair, got myself (well, shoplifted) some Bonne Bell lip gloss and Bain de Soleil (for the St. Tropez tan), and saved up my lawn-mowing money for a yellow velour bikini. That accomplished, I thought I was one foxy lady.

Nothing could have been further from the truth, and here is where I was introduced to the great paradox of being female in the modern world. I may have possessed a mass of curlywavyfrizzy hair, big shoulders and hips, and strong legs and not-big-enough-tits, but I had a small waist, skin that tanned beautifully, and dimples. Especially with my newly glossed lips and bronzed complexion, I thought I looked hot. But whatever beauty I possessed—and without even looking at an old picture I can assure you it was the innate radiance of the young and healthy—it was not the *right* kind of beauty. You know the one I mean—the one that is always impossible to obtain, manage, and maintain, regardless of the era.

My mother was aware of both the prevailing beauty standards of the day, and the degree to which I failed to measure up to them. In sixth grade, we were required to be measured and weighed by the school nurse. I was five foot eight, the second tallest girl in the class. That I weighed 115 pounds mattered not. I was clearly on my way to becoming an unlovable colossus. This calamity was no match for *Seventeen* magazine, to which my mother had already subscribed me. She panicked and took me straight to my pediatrician. The unacceptability of my glorious, healthy female body required medical intervention.

"What can we *do*?" she asked Dr. Swift (his real name). "What if she gets taller?"

"You could try giving her coffee," he said. As if I wasn't standing right there.

"What about cigarettes? I read where smoking could stunt a person's growth."

Dr. Swift, who was known to light up in the exam room on occasion, pondered the idea before suggesting we all just "wait and see."

At the time, I was merely confused: weren't cigarettes a grown-up thing, like taxes? It wasn't until sophomore year in high school when we saw a film in Health about how smoking could kill you that I put two and two together: I was so monstrously tall that my mother and my fucking *doctor* thought the risk of lung cancer was worth it if it would shave off an inch of my adult height. I never took up smoking, by the way. I was, and still am, five foot eight.

Worse than being too tall and flat-chested was my insistence on "carrying on," my mother's catchall term for being boisterous, competitive, obsessed by "cockamamie" topics (hummingbirds, Cleopatra, the French Revolution), and incapable of sitting still with a pleasant smile on my face. It was clear that not only my appearance, but also my personality needed a makeover.

My mother knew I was smart and determined. She also knew that unmitigated, these traits would drive away the men of the world, like the Godzilla monster terrorizing the tiny citizens of Tokyo. However—happy news!—I *could* leverage my intelligence and drive to completely remake myself. I could discipline myself to appear less than, which would increase my attractiveness to boys. I could transform myself into an innocuous female clever enough to hide her intelligence and savvy enough to know the exact moment when, in the company of boys or men, to become charming and ineffectual. I could "watch my figure" and read books like *How to Get a Teen-Age Boy and What to Do with Him When You Get Him*, which my mother thoughtfully gave to me in my Easter basket after her unilateral decision that I didn't need any more yellow Peeps, jelly beans, or hollow chocolate bunnies. I recall feeling distressed and frustrated by this. My mother's message was clear: my True Self was unlovable. Boys were drawn to a very specific kind of girl, and only with a great deal of work could I fashion myself into that girl. And she wasn't wrong. No one asked me to the eighth-grade dance, and my crushes of that year all went unrequited.

My mother didn't have much to say about feminism. She was in her late thirties when the second wave crashed on the shores of our conservative California suburb, and however much she enjoyed having a credit card in her own name, she still believed the best way a girl could get ahead was by marrying well. She was interested in style, in her suburban middle-class way—she had a staggering collection of dangly earrings—and fully understood the quiet, doe-eyed appeal of Julie Barnes, the character played by the exquisite Peggy Lipton on *The Mod Squad*. She completely got the allure of Joni Mitchell, the long

flaxen hair, fetching overbite, skinny arms, and baby voice.*
She was smart enough, my mother, not to try to squeeze me
into the housewife mold she'd squeezed herself into as if it
were a longline girdle.

Even so, her mandate was clear: that my goal in life, the thing
to which I was supposed to devote my time and energy, was
becoming a human being who lived to please everyone around
her. All this self-improvement was not for me, per se, but for
the reactions it would elicit in others—not just boys, although
they made up the main audience, but also teachers, coaches,
friends and their parents, and the boss at the dog grooming
place where I worked at sixteen who liked to rest his hand on
my ass.

I was too much and never enough. Too much curiosity and
stubbornness. Not enough bubbly receptivity. Too tall. Not
dainty ever, or at all. Too me. Not enough Julie and Joni. My
mother was disappointed when I wasn't invited to the big
school dances, or when, at teacher conferences, my American
history teacher Mrs. Quigley said I could be "a bit outspoken"
in class. To further break her heart, I was voted Most $@#^*!
in our senior class, loosely translated as Most Infuriating, our
school's moniker for class clown. It seemed that no amount of
hair ironing or dieting or pretending to be interested in any

---

* My mom had no opinion about Mitchell's obvious musical genius, which
breaks my heart a little.

banal remark that fell out of a cute boy's mouth made a difference. My snarky, willful, rambunctious self would find a way to express herself, and thus ruin my life.

By sixteen, I felt perpetually at odds with myself. To be myself meant failing at culturally sanctioned femininity; to succeed at culturally sanctioned femininity meant failing myself. I felt alone in this ongoing anguish, but I was not. As I've grown up and older, I've discovered that many, if not most, smart, competent women possess a similar story.

Until very recently, self-improvement hasn't really been much of a practical concern for men. Cogitating on how a man might improve himself used to be an occupation of the educated and the wealthy. Plato lounged on his thinking pillow in ancient Greece and advised his students: *for a man to conquer himself is the first and noblest of all victories.* The man in question here is literally a man, not the old-school pronoun that also included women. Marcus Aurelius, Confucius, Descartes, Benjamin Franklin, and all the other guys who spent their lives pondering how we should then live, were addressing men. (Women, less valued than livestock, were off sewing curtains for the menstrual hut.)

But, for the most part, men improve themselves by gaining skills. They are rarely pressed into completely retooling their personalities to succeed in a way appropriate to their gender. Consider my husband's upbringing. When I asked him about his experience of self-improvement as a child, the first thing I had to do was *clarify* what I meant by self-improvement. This pretty much answered my question. He was born in 1975, the eldest of four, and his mother thought he was a princeling. She enjoyed his company. She taught him to ride a horse and together they took tap-dancing lessons. His father, a busy real estate attorney, worked long hours. However, he did coach Little League. The only thing my husband recalls having been ordered to do by his father is choke up on the bat and get in front of the ball, standard coaching directives. Regarding school, he was told he needed to "focus," which frustrated both him and his parents; at fourteen he was diagnosed with ADD. What was utterly lacking in his experience was the ongoing drama of who he was. He wasn't subscribed to any advertising-heavy magazines devoted to teaching him about how to be a perfect boy. When he was in sixth grade, he was short and chubby, but his parents assumed he'd grow out of it, and lo and behold, he did. He was pressured to do things better, but there was no expectation that he would completely remake his essential self to make himself more likable.

Fast-forward to 2020, where men, unless they're among the very rich, are now feeling a lot of self-defeating feelings that women have long lived with—that they're not good enough, that they need fixing. They are being marketed to like mad, and so, like women, are now experiencing the anxiety-producing pressure of self-improvement.

Scroll through the comments on novelist Jessica Knoll's *New York Times* op-ed "Smash the Wellness Industry: Why Are So

Many Smart Women Falling for Its Harmful, Pseudoscientific Claims?" and you will see modern men possess their own brand of distress.

Emanuel from St. Louis sums it up nicely: "If you think that men aren't self-conscious about their bodies and are not victims of the wellness industry, you are very wrong. Men see male models and movie stars with lean muscular bodies and feel inadequacy just as women do. Though I do not know how women feel in comparison to men on this issue, I can say that if men seem to not worry about their bodies, it's because it's a very 'unmanly' thing to complain about."

In *Kids These Days: Human Capital and the Making of Millennials*, Malcolm Harris's defense of that beleaguered generation, it becomes clear why men are starting to embrace the fantasy of self-improvement. A millennial himself, Harris points out that even though people born between 1980 and 2000 are the world's most educated and skilled generation, the market can't accommodate them. It is no longer enough for a guy to show up to a job interview in an ironed shirt with a proofread résumé and a can-do attitude and expect to be hired at a wage commensurate with his education. In the gig economy, all those enriching math camps and Mandarin classes mean nothing. One of the fallouts of life under late-stage capitalism, where the world's top twenty-six billionaires (collectively worth $1.4 trillion) own more than the poorest 3.8 billion people, or roughly half the world's population, is that men are now feeling a pressure to fix themselves in a way that looks very familiar to the gender that has been pushing the self-improvement rock uphill since middle school. Welcome to the club, guys!

Marketers and advertisers, always ahead of the curve, are right there, offering guys a competitive edge. Men are pummeled with messages about "personal optimization," how to be more productive, more organized, more stoic (stoicism is very hot right now), all in the pursuit of You 2.0. A January 2019 article in *Men's Health* recommended that to improve themselves men should set (more) goals, learn something new (by watching YouTube tutorials), make a rainy-day fund, hang out with friends, and "reorganize a bit." Intermittent fasting has been adopted by dudes, and more men than ever are displaying signs of eating disorders.

Depending on their proclivities, men are going vegan and training for ultramarathons, or awaking at 4:00 a.m. and organizing the shit out of every minute of their lives to be more productive. Those who haven't given up, retiring to their mom's basement to pwn noobs* on Overwatch or anyone who has it better on social media, are now forced to improve themselves if they want to get ahead, or even tread water.

I asked a politically minded friend what she thinks of when she hears the word *patriarchy*, and she said she sometimes imag-

---

* Video-game speak for when a skilled player annihilates an inexperienced player or newbie, also known as "noob." The skilled player, temporarily deranged by his awesomeness and eager to brag about his prowess, often mistypes *own* as *pwn*—*p* being next to *o* on the keyboard.

ines a gigantic, windowless Las Vegas hotel conference room where powerful men assemble and make decisions that benefit only other men. I mentioned that famous John Trumbull painting of the signing of the Declaration of Independence, where wealthy, well-educated, landowning white men stood around looking pensive in their white wigs, while crafting a document that didn't include the rights of women and slaves. She laughed and said, "Exactly!"

But the concept of patriarchy in 2020 needs some tweaking. I fear we've stereotyped patriarchy to everyone's disadvantage but the ultrarich.* Patriarchy isn't the monolith we presume it is. It's not a rocky cliff against which the evolving waves of feminism crash and disperse. I'm pro–smashing the patriarchy, but only insofar as it means smashing every injustice issuing from the poison fruit of old institutions guaranteed to keep money and power in the hands of the very wealthy. Most of these institutions serve not only privileged white men, but also their women. Let us never forget that 52 percent of white women who voted in the 2016 presidential election, according to exit polls, voted for Donald Trump.

A simple survey of the regular joes in your life is more illuminating than a thousand think pieces about how patriarchy is going for the 99 percent. Wages have stagnated, good jobs are scarce, and forget about gratifying long-term careers with

---

* I vote for a new term, the *ultraricharchy.*

reasonable benefits. How many men do you know who have multiple jobs? How many have side hustles, a trendy name for what is just more low-paid work, performed at odd hours? During the writing of this book, I conducted an informal survey of Lyft drivers. One hundred percent had other jobs. My husband is a computer network engineer who works as a "consultant." He's available to his clients all hours of the day and night.* He has had to cut his hourly rate to stay competitive, and obviously has no benefits, including health insurance. His side hustle is as a fix-it man.

I know it's hideously unfashionable to have any sympathy for white men, but the Trump presidency *has* made things worse for these lower-rung stewards of the patriarchy. His monumental tax cuts favor only businesses and the wealthy. Everyone else, including millions of other men, can suck it. Men have been sold out by their brethren, and their remaining option, after blaming women, people of color, and members of the LGBTQIA community, is to improve themselves. It doesn't occur to them, poor darlings, that the perpetrators of this mess, the masterminds behind the collapse of decent jobs with modest benefits and the increase in the already astronomical costs of education and health care, are *other men.* Either that or "bros before hos" is simply baked into their DNA, and if that's the case we're pretty much doomed.

---

* A recent frantic 2:00 a.m. text: "I can't open my email!!!!"

Thus, to succeed under late-stage capitalism, men must improve themselves by becoming lean, mean machines of self-optimizing productivity. They must learn the ten rules of success and the seven habits of highly effective people, successfully embrace change and change their mindsets, identify their self-sabotaging beliefs, and overcome self-imposed limitations. It would be nice if they would also trim their toenails, but real change takes time. As you can tell, I've now exhausted my empathy for men. I've said yeah, no, not happening to pretending I have an endless supply. Back to our regular programing.

All this is to say that while twenty-first-century men have joined us in the complicated dance of self-improvery, their steps are much easier to master. They want to go for something, they go for it. They want to get better at something, they try to get better. Whether they succeed is something else. They want to up their game at the office? They work to up their game at the office. They don't have to mask their ambition, or that they're angling for that promotion and the corner office. Absent in their quest for self-betterment are the paradoxes at the heart of female self-improvery that ensure we are always simmering with confusion and self-recrimination.

For women, self-improvement is a damned-if-you-do-damned-if-you-don't conundrum that must be negotiated with the strategic powers of Alexander the Great. A woman must always be working to perfect her physical self, while also trying to figure out how to make life easier for everyone around her. She is expected to do this with a spring in her step and a song in her heart, without conflicting emotions or a bad attitude. If she starts feeling a little murderous, there is a meditation app for that, another SoulCycle class, hormone replacement therapy, or that old stand-by, retail therapy. (We feel especially better when we're buying things to improve ourselves, which is why buying a $200 monthlong package at a yoga studio doesn't feel like spending real money.)

However, if a woman spends too much time improving a skill for her own pleasure, or in her own self-interest—or even for her *job*—if she is unapologetically competent, smart, and ambitious, she risks becoming unlikable, a disastrous turn of events. Look no further than the adventures of Hillary Clinton, easily the most despised woman in America in 2016, whose only crime was having man-size ambition, something she did nothing to conceal. Or at least not enough.

To be sure, men running for public office are also judged on their likability, but like self-improvement, they're judged on different merits. In 2004 George W. Bush was "the guy you'd want to have a beer with" presidential candidate because he was affable and a little dorky and looked like he would always be the one *buying* the beers. In 2008, candidate Mitt Romney became unlikable when it was revealed that in 1983, heading off on a family vacation, he strapped his Irish setter, Seamus, to the roof of the car in a pet carrier for the twelve-hour drive. Romney's lame explanation that "my dog likes fresh air" added tone-deaf idiot to animal abuser on his rap sheet of public opinion. But even though we are a nation of dog lovers, Romney's political career only temporarily tanked. In 2018, he was elected to the Senate. There is no likability "trap" for men; they earn their unlikability fair and square. After which they take a long vacation somewhere out West, work on their tan, then present themselves as if nothing untoward had happened.

Joan C. Williams, in a *New York Times* op-ed called "How Women Can Escape the Likability Trap: Powerful Women Know How to Flip Feminine Stereotypes to Their Advantage," underscored this depressing quandary by offering up a "set of strategies" to escape being disliked. She advocates "thinking of femininity as a tool kit."[*] She suggests using "softeners" while negotiating a salary.[†] Williams is a no-nonsense pragmatist in a girl's-gotta-do-what-a-girl's-gotta-do fashion that neatly sidesteps the issue of whether powerful women should use their power to effect change, but the larger point is this: the better women get at what they do, the more they improve, the better they must also be at not appearing to be too good at what they do. It's at the heart of the double bind of a life devoted to self-improvement: we must not be too much, while hamster-wheeling our effort to be enough.

---

[*] As if women haven't been doing *that* since the dawn of time.

[†] Not related to laundry, "softeners" are used to ask-without-asking, and were employed with great success by thoroughbred Sheryl Sandberg to squeeze a raise from her boss, archdweeb Mark Zuckerberg.

How are we too much? We are too complicated, too opin-ionated, too angry, too emotional. "Too smart for your own good" is surely an observation reserved only for women. Celeb-rities with fan bases rivaling the population of a small country still possess legions of haters. In *Too Fat, Too Slutty, Too Loud: The Rise and Reign of the Unruly Woman*, BuzzFeed culture writer Anne Helen Petersen surveys ten female icons and the backlash they endure as penance for disobeying the dictates of traditional femininity. Madonna is too old, Serena Williams is too strong, novelist Jennifer Weiner is too loud, etc. Proof, as if we needed it, that even (maybe especially) women who possess money, power, fame, and better-than-average looks—everything Western consumer culture considers the golden tickets to happiness—are despised for pushing boundaries. Pe-tersen writes, "To be an unruly woman today is to oscillate between the postures of fearlessness and self-doubt, between listening to the voices that tell a woman she is *too much* and one's own, whispering and yelling *I am already enough, and always have been.*"

How are we never enough? That's easy—not pretty enough, slim enough, sexy enough, feminine enough. As second-wave feminist and author Susan Brownmiller noted in the 1980s, "Every woman is a female impersonator." Performative fem-ininity is a role, as unnatural to the gender to which it is ascribed as it is to the drag queens who've made it an art form. And still we persist on beating ourselves up, and giving far too many fucks, when we fail to live up to this impossible ideal.

There is an exception: the only time we're permitted to be too much is when we're also more than beautiful enough, slender enough, and stylish enough, which only happens on TV lawyer shows.

Suits, the long-running television show that premiered in 2011, is about one of New York's "top law firms." It costars Meghan Markle in her pre–Duchess of Sussex days and features a bevy of legal geniuses (Harvard law!) who are also exquisite beauties living in an eternal state of red-carpet readiness. Jessica Pearson, played by Gina Torres, a named partner, is a Harvard graduate, legal genius, and nervy strategist. She is allowed her fictional badassery because she is absolutely ravishing in her designer ensembles, rocking full makeup and a mane of carefully styled hair. She is never seen to do a moment's work, but rather slinks around the office as if she's on the catwalk. Sometimes she perches on the edge of a desk holding a file folder.

Striving to be pretty, thin, and hot enough, while at the same time working to quash every personality trait that makes you feel like your True Self, makes *you* interesting, and in turn makes life interesting and confers upon you the individuality that we all worship in men but find suspect in women, is a recipe for nonstop distress and anxiety. And how are we advised to relieve our distress and quell our anxiety? By "improving" ourselves, doubling down on our efforts to be prettier, thinner, hotter while doing more to smooth our too muchness— exercising to the point of exhaustion, self-medicating with tequila (made from agave, and thus almost a green smoothie), and downloading a new personality-management app.

Not only is there no finish line, but the perfect woman-self we're seeking is also a moving target. Jia Tolentino, writing about Naomi Wolf's work in *Trick Mirror*, sums up the perpetual motion machine of a life of self-improvement thus: "In 1991, Naomi Wolf wrote, in *The Beauty Myth*, about the peculiar fact that beauty requirements have escalated as women's subjugation has decreased. It's as if our culture has mustered an immune-system response to continue breaking the fever of gender equality— as if some deep patriarchal logic has made it that women need to achieve ever-higher levels of beauty to make up for the fact that we are no longer economically and legally dependent on men. One waste of time has been traded for another."

As I was writing and rewriting this section, something began to strike a false note. The sentiment *feels* accurate, but it doesn't really hold up under scrutiny. More likely, the impulse to achieve ever-higher levels of beauty is related not to some secret cabal of beauty arbitrators, but to the bombardment of ads every time we check our phones, ads promoting the usual panic-inducing state that we don't measure up, and that have nothing to do with who we are and everything to do with some corporation's bottom line. And who is this mighty invisible jury legislating these acceptable levels of beauty? When Tolentino anthropomorphizes culture, giving it an immune system, or refers to "deep patriarchal logic," which, again, alludes to some invisible, powerful judiciary hearing the cases of individual women and meting out punishment, who is she talking about?

In op-eds, think pieces, personal essays, manifestos, and mighty social media screeds, writers sling around a lot of *they*s, as if culture, society, the patriarchy, the FLEBers, the Lululemon moms—choose your oppressors—are standing armies that exist only to keep our self-esteem low and our compulsive desire to improve ourselves high. Catchy phrases identifying recent trends involving and perpetuated by "them" are coined by journalists to garner clicks. Often, the journalists are pressed into inflating a random idea they pulled out of their asses at three a.m. (not that I would know anything about this) into what sounds like a legitimate sociological or psychological paradigm by an editor, who in turn has been pressured by the money people. I don't know who coined the likability trap, but it's only a trap if you think it's a trap. In France, where I now live, women who strive to be likable are thought to be "uninteresting," so it's far from being a universal dilemma.

And let us recall that aside from our nearest and dearest, few people think about us deeply enough to gauge the degree to which they like us. This is not to say people aren't making snap judgments and projecting their own insecurities on us like mad, but as I discussed in chapter 1, most people aren't paying close attention to us, and if they are, it's to determine whether we're paying attention to them. Essayist Alain de Botton, self-described philosopher of everyday life and cofounder of London's The School of Life, wrote a lengthy Facebook post on the topic. He describes the shock of realizing, usually sometime in late adolescence, that we don't matter to all but a very few people. All the strangers who smiled at us when we were children and gave us free lollipops, those teachers who applauded our mediocre efforts and were invested in our doing better—those people are gone and that time of our life is over. It's such a brutal lesson we don't believe it. We still go to parties, and stand around with a glass of mineral water, sure people are talking about how we're trying to get sober or lose weight. We give a presentation at work and worry for a week that everyone noticed we stumbled over the names of our team. We go to the doctor and feel a rush of shame when we step on the scale.

To absorb the truth of the world's indifference, de Botton suggests a thought exercise to challenge ourselves to see how much we pay attention to others. Of the experience, he writes, "Imagine that we're in a lift, standing next to someone on our way to the twentieth floor. They know we disapprove of their choice of jacket. They know they should have picked another one and that they look silly and pinched in this one. But we haven't noticed the jacket. In fact, we haven't noticed they were born—or that one day they will die. We're just worrying about how our partner responded when we mentioned our mother's cold to them last night."

He hastens to reassure his readers that he knows we're not uncaring and irresponsible. If someone is drowning, we jump in. If a friend is sobbing in distress, we pay attention and try to comfort her. When our report is due on the boss's desk at noon, you can bet that she's paying attention (because the report affects *her*). But unless the situation demands it, we pay attention to ourselves and our own lives. De Botton ends the post with an interesting twist. Not only is it ultimately freeing to realize no one is paying attention, but in gratitude we should pay the liberation forward by not paying attention to others. Which, conveniently, removes the temptation to judge or otherwise shame them, and releases them from feeling like they must do something to improve themselves. Everybody wins.

I will never for one second blame a woman for being unable to manage her self-talk in a way that uplifts her, but there is a lot of power in calling bullshit. What if we just stopped thinking we were too much and never enough? What if we shrugged in the face of so-called higher levels of beauty? What if we retired the whole paradigm of the likability trap like a threadbare pair of yoga pants with a hole in the crotch? What if, the next time someone said, or intimated, that you were "too" something, you just laughed? What if, instead of taking that person seriously, you decided they were too stupid or, if you're kinder than I am, were simply misguided and thus wrong? What if you looked in the mirror and said, "I am pretty"? Full stop. Just typing that, I feel like a fucking revolutionary.

I remember a conversation I had with my mother the summer between high school and college. We had just come from a doctor's appointment and were on our way to the mall to begin shopping for clothes for, as she called it, my new adventure. I had been accepted to USC, where my father had gone to college, and where she hoped I would meet boys who, she said, were more our ilk. "You're going to be able to make a fresh start," she said. I had watched enough TV to know that people who made fresh starts were usually on the lam. They'd robbed a bank or had a baby "out of wedlock" or in some other way ruined their lives and brought shame down upon the heads of their well-meaning mothers.

In my memory, I sighed and looked out the window at our sun-blasted suburb. The poisonous pink-and-white oleander, the lush palm trees in which roof rats nested. I was irritated. She could take her ilk—which I heard as *elk*—and shove it. "Fuck you," I said in my head. I remember that part clear as day.

I mark that drive to the mall as both the beginning and the end of my teenage rebellion. A few weeks later something unforeseen happened. My mother was diagnosed with an aggressive form of brain cancer. Four months after an unsuccessful surgery to excise the tumor, while I was away at school, she slipped into a coma and died. I'd last seen her alive on my eighteenth birthday. Even then this struck me as ridiculously symbolic. I imagined that she took one look at me on that day, realized I was never going to be the girl she wanted me to be, and gave up. It took a decade of therapy for me to accept that I had not killed her by failing to improve myself.

CHAPTER 4

Your Best Self Is Like an Imaginary Beloved

No need to hurry. No need to sparkle. No need to be anybody but oneself.

—Virginia Woolf, *A Room of One's Own*

What is our best self? Do we even know? Or is it one of those terms we throw around with confidence, even though we're not exactly clear what we mean by it? We know becoming our best self can't mean obtaining perfection, because that's impossible. Or is it? I suspect we secretly suppose that becoming the perfect woman is possible if we just fully commit ourselves to the process and think super positive thoughts and get up an hour earlier to do an enriching thing. Why else do we still yearn to look like celebrities whose perfect photographs we are well aware have been photoshopped?

I have some bad news. This so-called best self—not to be confused with ourselves at our best; more about that in a few pages—is a mythological creature who runs in the same crowd as our imaginary beloved. If you've never had one, the imaginary beloved is your soul mate, the person of your dreams who doesn't exist but who nevertheless thrills and consoles you. One contributor to Thought Catalog wrote about her imaginary boyfriend: "He would be smart, tall, and romantic. He would be an excellent writer, his hands would be strong, he would know how to cook me a perfect meal, he would be sensitive and he would travel with me." My imaginary boyfriend, whom I concocted in eighth grade and revived again my freshman year in college, was named Rocky. He was a surfer intellectual who lived in Santa Barbara. He had a shy smile and a hank of sun-streaked hair that hung over green eyes. His favorite book was *Thus Spoke Zarathustra*, and there may have also been a puka shell necklace involved.

The advantage of having an imaginary beloved is that they care about what we think, don't text when we talk, and bring us hot and sour soup from the farther-away but infinitely better Chinese place when we're sick. They treat us with respect. Imagining the relationship with the imaginary beloved is a creative exercise: what kind of person would love me, and how would they love me, just as I am?

Our best self is just as fantastical, but from the day we start wondering what we can do to be as pretty as our favorite Disney princess, we're conditioned to believe that seeking to be our best self is not just a doable goal, but the primary goal of our lives. It's only when we get a little older that we discover that our best self is a chimera.

In 1972, English painter and art critic John Berger published *Ways of Seeing*, adapted from his popular BBC television series, which aired the same year and demystified the work of the art critic. First and foremost a primer on how to look at paintings, *Ways of Seeing* contained a section that discussed the objectification of women in works of art. Essentially, men watch women and women watch themselves being watched. Second-wave feminism effectively repurposed Berger's theory, and in 1975, film critic Laura Mulvey would coin the term *male gaze* to describe the way the world, including the women in it, is viewed through the lens of the heterosexual male. In the visual arts, this applied to an unseen trinity of men: the man making the picture, the men viewing the picture, and also the men in the tableau, looking at and evaluating the women in the picture.

For the purposes of figuring out how to swear off self-improvement, I'm more interested in Berger's idea that women have been trained to watch themselves as a matter of survival. We must literally watch ourselves, and watch ourselves being watched, because for millennia we've been forced to function within a society created by and for men. How we come across to men has determined the quality of our lives. "A woman must continually watch herself," Berger writes. "She is almost continually accompanied by her own image of herself. While she is walking across a room or while she is weeping at the death of her father, she can scarcely avoid envisaging herself walking or weeping. From earliest childhood, she has been taught and persuaded to survey herself continually. *And so she comes to consider the* surveyor *and the* surveyed *within her as the two constituent yet always distinct elements of her identity as a woman.*" (Italics mine.)

I didn't learn about John Berger and the male gaze until graduate school, five years after my mother's death. By then it was the 1980s and already Berger's viewpoints were being debated. What about gays and lesbians? What about the female gaze? The night of the afternoon of my mother's funeral, I drove back to USC and took an oceanography midterm. As it happened, I had envisaged what I looked like not weeping. I remained unemotional, stony-faced in my burgundy prairie-style Gunne Sax dress—I refused to wear black. I never saw a counselor. Six months after my mother died my father rekindled a relationship with his college sweetheart, signaling that it was time we moved on.

During those years, I was very aware of watching myself, of containing two women. The Surveyor made sure the Surveyed appeared to be cheerful, fun-loving, and up for anything! The Surveyed attended class, dutifully partied, developed obligatory crushes on boys whose last names she never bothered learning. The Surveyor swung between feeling guilty that

she'd killed her mother because she was such a disappointment, and rage that her mother, so frustrated at having to deal
with a girl who could not, would not, improve herself, had no
recourse but to manifest an aggressive brain tumor and try
her luck in the next world.

To the therapist I saw fifteen years later, I would describe that
time as if I were living inside a glass tube. I could see people but
couldn't touch them. They could see me but didn't try to touch
me. Decades later I came upon a more perfect description. Heidi
Julavits, writing in her memoir *The Folded Clock*, described her
experience at a prestigious writing retreat in Italy. One day,
she ventured out to see Piero's Madonna. The contemplation of
the Madonna, according to the "head pilgrim" on the visit, could
change the outcome of your life. But the painting was difficult
to see beneath not one but two layers of glass, like "trying to
see a jam jar inside of an aquarium," a description that Julavits
then used to describe her time at the retreat, which she had
been unable to enjoy.

I gasped when I read that description. That was me. I had
been inside that jam jar, inside that aquarium. Once, I got
stupid drunk and went with a Sigma Chi to his bedroom. He
didn't touch me. I walked on a Mexican beach at midnight
with a guy I'd met in a bar. I hitchhiked in Morocco. In Mar-
rakesh, I went back with a guy to his room at 2:00 a.m. We
slept side by side in his bed like siblings. Nothing bad happened. Nothing good happened. My guardian angel was working overtime, but while I was engaging in this stupid risky

behavior, I felt safe, because I could feel people distancing themselves from me.

No matter how hard the Surveyor worked to improve the Surveyed in those days (fad diets, aerobics, weekly face masks, a deep investigation into the best mascara), I remained unlikable. Or that was how it seemed to me then, thus proving that once again, my mother had been right. Much later, I would realize that we were all just kids, and no one knew what to say to someone who'd suffered such a horrifying loss.

Kathryn Schulz, writing in *New York* magazine in 2013, describes this same bifurcated self: "Let us call it the master theory of self-help. It goes like this: somewhere below or above or beyond the part of you that is struggling with weight loss or procrastination or whatever your particular problem might be, there is another part of you that is immune to that problem and capable of solving it for the rest of you. In other words, this master theory is fundamentally dualist. It posits, at a minimum, two selves: one that needs a kick in the ass and one that is capable of kicking."

The Surveyed is the one who needs the kick in the ass, and the Surveyor is the one to do it. But the Surveyed is someone we've manufactured, according to the female ideal of the time, and the one who becomes our best self, our imaginary beloved. Our Surveyor is most likely to be closer to our true, unvarnished self.

I imagine serious, competent Surveyor Karen hard at work in black T-shirt, baggy jeans, yellow reflective vest, and orange hard hat, gazing through her telescopic machine at shiny, people-pleasing Surveyed Karen. The jeans worn by Surveyed Karen are flattering, overthought, and overpriced, incorporating some sort of trademarked butt-lifting, tummy-flattening technology. Her black blouse is silky, figure-defining while also providing discreet coverage for her much-despised armpit fat. Her hair has been dyed, shampooed, conditioned, treated with a hair mask to encourage shine, air-dried, and tossed like a salad with an expensive tonic designed to preserve her natural waves. (It costs $250 every six weeks.) She wears a foundation that is supposed to give her skin a dewy sheen. An expensive concealer hides her age spots but not her freckles. The aesthetician who gives her monthly facials assured her that freckles are "young-ifying." Surveyed is wearing a maximizing lip-plumping lip gloss in raspberry. She smiles, even when she is alone; Surveyor has done research, educating Surveyed in the power of smiling, the way it puts you in a better mood, while also toning the muscles of the face.

Body dysmorphic disorder (BDD) is defined as an obsessive preoccupation with some aspect of our bodies—hair, skin, nose, chest, and stomach are most common. BDD entered the *Diagnostic and Statistical Manual of Mental Disorders* (DSM) in 1987 and is believed to be on the obsessive-compulsive disorder spectrum. It's been described as "the distress of imagined ugliness." Those who suffer from BDD focus on their perceived flaws for much of their waking hours. Muscle dysmorphia, suffered mostly by men, is the excessive belief that your body is too underdeveloped and skinny. It entered the DSM in 2013, as a subcategory of BDD.

I'd like to suggest a new addition to the dysmorphia family: best-self dysmorphia. The primary symptom of best-self dysmorphia disorder (BSDD) is the constant feeling that however "good" we are, we are never enough. The Surveyor, always chasing the best self, is never satisfied with the achievements of the Surveyed.

Whatever our goals, they could be better. If we've achieved those goals, we realize they should have been bigger and more ambitious. Whatever our mood, it could be more pleasant. However productive we are, we could be more productive. Our spiritual practice could be more spiritual. Our relationships could be more relation-y. Our thoughts could be more focused and positive, because the Universe is always listening, so every musing must always be intentional and pure of heart, or we risk not receiving the things we feel we need to make us happy.

Do not mistake BSDD with the healthy human desire to take care of ourselves and do the things necessary to maintain a healthy body. I am not suggesting that we shouldn't eat right, exercise, take time to rest and reflect, and all the other things I know you already know are good for you. I'm also all for self-actualization: indeed, learning what to say yes to, and what to say fuck it all about, is a component of self-growth.

BSDD is not self-actualization, though it often wears it as a disguise. BSDD is that crazy-making conviction that no matter what you've achieved, how much you're loved, how much you have, you need to be doing more, or something different, to assure continued achievement, love, acquisition, and happiness. The food on the BSDD sufferer's plate could always be greener and leaner. If it was once considered an inedible noxious weed but has now been revealed to be a superfood, she could not be happier. BSDD also features a strong component of body dissatisfaction. She could always be fitter, eat better, take better care of her skin, have more hair where she's supposed to have more hair and less hair where she's supposed to have less, and look chic rather than misguided in those giant baggy linen dresses that are currently all the rage.

My friend Maggie suffers from BSDD tendencies, and she's the first to admit it. Maggie has a functional marriage, a job in tech she likes well enough, and a nice house in a nice neighborhood. Her husband is not preoccupied by his phone, cooks a few nights a week, and remembers all the important anniversaries. The house has a walk-in pantry and a sunroom surrounded by fig trees. She wants for nothing that any of us who love her can see; many people do love her, and to my knowledge no one thinks she needs to be better than she already is. She tends to finish your sentences, drinks too much and gets weepy three days after her nutty mother visits, borrows books then claims they were hers to start with, and brags too much about how woke her son is compared to other sons. In short: her best self is her real self and is just as flawed as the rest of us, and no one holds it against her.

She is, however, obsessed with her weight, which is average for her height. Still, she felt she could lose twenty pounds. She yearned to fit into a pair of cutoffs she found in a box in the attic that she wore when she was eleven, or some crazy-ass nonsense. She went paleo and lost twenty pounds. She became slightly mad with her rapid weight loss (as one does), started running, upped her daily mileage, then blew out her knee. During her recovery, she discovered salted caramel ice cream and a Netflix show with seven or eight seasons and gained it all back. She was once again at her average weight, and back to being unable to fit into the clothes she wore as a tween. To manage her self-loathing, she tried meditation, then missed a few mornings, then felt guilty. She felt guilty for feeling guilty. It's meditation, not trauma surgery, she tried to tell herself. She descended into a bad period of lacerating self-hatred.

There was no convincing her that anyone who has an active life risks getting injured. Bad stuff happens. And when it does, sometimes we just freak out and find comfort where we can. We retreat to a place that feels good, even if it's not good for us, and lick our wounds. Or an ice-cream cone. It's frustrating, but it doesn't merit the searing self-loathing, self-doubt, and despair we all feel when we've fallen off our best self–seeking wagon.

Emma, another friend, is trying to get pregnant. Every month, when her period comes, she thinks: if I would just be able to quit coffee, wine, sugar, gluten, and dairy, and be mindful and get more exercise, more sleep, and drink more water, and focus on empowering my lady plumbing to get with it, I would get pregnant. She believes in the power of the mind-body connection, and when she feels stuck in her head (all the time; like so many of us she's strapped to her laptop and phone), she feels like she's falling down on the job. She's aware that she's trying to have agency over something beyond her control, but it's also been drilled into her that everything is her responsibility. She believes the mind-body connection isn't a democracy, but a dictatorship, where the mind gives the orders. To accept there is sometimes plain old bad luck, or situations over which we have no control, is tantamount to quitting. And Emma's best self doesn't quit.

She knows she's being hard on herself, but to give up on being an improved version of herself, in Emma's mind—in so many of our minds—is synonymous with being a failure. "I know I should be the woman who juices and goes to yoga, declutters, and has a growing 401(k), but instead I wind up watching TV and eating a doughnut," she says. In her voice, you can hear her disappointment and despair. Emma is a fantastic baker and could easily open a business selling one thing: her mouthwatering apple spice cinnamon doughnuts. For the record, if those are the doughnuts she's eating, it makes complete sense. She would be insane not to sit around eating those doughnuts and binge-watching *Stranger Things*.

The last time I talked to Emma she had just attended a women's summit sponsored by Princeton, her alma mater. All the featured speakers and keynotes, women at the top of their game in the top of their fields, women who've launched companies, litigated landmark cases, patented forward-thinking technology that will save the planet, married well, birthed well, are raising handsome and exemplary children, manage to maintain homes with white sofas and black dogs, all while rocking artfully torn size 2 skinny jeans and a cashmere sweater, felt they didn't measure up. Over goblets of dry rosé, they talked about feeling like frauds, and about all the ways in which they still were not doing their best.

Emma said, "Isn't that horrifying? I mean, all those accomplished women who still think they're not good enough."

"Yeah, you're one of them," I said with love.

"Fuck off, so are you," she said. (Also with love.)

She was right, of course.

Best self is a creation, as we've established. Best self is a collaboration between the culture and our Surveyor. The culture makes its impossible demands, always shifting with the times, and the Surveyor presses the Surveyed to keep up.

Culture says, "Your hair may be straight, but it isn't silky enough." Surveyor tells Surveyed, "You should get a keratin treatment, stat!" Culture says, "You may be thin, but do you wear a size 0?" Surveyor tells Surveyed, "You should cut out bananas. They're the most fattening fruit. Also, you should up your workout from forty-five minutes a day to ninety." Culture asks, "Are you making sure you are available to tend to everyone in your family 24/7, with a smile on your chemically peeled face?" Surveyor tells Surveyed, "You should get better at time management and find some happy-all-the-time mantra to keep resentment at bay."

Best self is a very powerful-seeming illusion. The iconic scene in *The Wizard of Oz* when Dorothy, the Scarecrow, the Tin Man, and the Lion finally reach the Emerald City and are granted an audience with the Wizard is an apt metaphor for seeing best self for who it is. Dorothy et al. stand trembling in the chamber before the Great Oz. His disembodied alien-looking head scowls at them from between pillars of fire. He roars and blusters, until Toto trots over and pulls aside a curtain, revealing the Wizard to be a harmless geezer pulling levers and shouting into a microphone. His power is pure sham.

What happens when we decide this crazy, futile pursuit of our best self isn't worth it anymore? Who are we when we say we're done with all that, and the world is going to have to accept us as we are? Who are we when we've had enough, and we're done playing by the rules, and the Surveyor stops ordering the Surveyed around, and they join forces?

The Self You Know to Be True in This Moment emerges. I'm going to call her True Self, to avoid using the completely out of control acronym, SYKTBTITM. It isn't a piece of cake to discern our True Self. Great thinkers since antiquity have spent entire lifetimes trying to define it. "I think, therefore I am," seventeenth-century philosopher René Descartes decided, sounding not at all certain. David Hume, tackling the definition a century later, declared the self to be a bundle of perceptions, "like links in a chain." (C+ effort, Mr. Hume.) Eastern thinkers sidestepped the definition and opted for aphorisms: "Knowing others is wisdom," wrote Lao Tzu in the fourth century BC. "Knowing yourself is enlightenment."

True Self, as I call her, is someone who has an inkling of her character traits, habits and behaviors, values and beliefs, personal preferences and tastes. There were times in my life when I was in such hot pursuit of best self, I lost track of what these qualities might be. Or worse, I thought they didn't matter. I thought True Self could be easily dismissed. I didn't respect her. I thought she was a nuisance, with her intelligence, her tendency to scoff at things over which other girls swooned, her love of mockery and practical jokes, her disinclination to be accommodating or pleasant.

Unlike best self, which is largely performative and presentational, True Self does not prioritize the way she is perceived by others. True Self dives in and responds, moment by moment, to what is going on around her and learns more about herself by the nature of these interactions. Mixing it up with other humans, diving wholeheartedly into new experiences, traveling—these are activities that reveal ourselves to ourselves.

To throw your lot in with True Self is to choose self-respect over the approval of others. I won't pretend that it doesn't take courage. As Joan Didion wrote in her 1961 *Vogue* essay "Self-Respect: Its Source, Its Power": ". . . people with self-respect exhibit a certain toughness, a kind of moral nerve; they display what was once called *character*, a quality which, although approved in the abstract, sometimes loses ground to other, more instantly negotiable virtues." The chief negotiable virtue for women, it seems to me, is convincing ourselves we're merely being flexible and open-minded when we succumb to the notion that consumer culture knows better about what it means to be a woman in the world than we do. Didion then goes on to say that character is the willingness to accept responsibility for our own life; relating it to self-improvement, we might extend that to mean responsibility for accepting our True Selves.

In 1999, when my dad was dying of lung cancer, I took care of him. I adored my dad, but my love for him didn't prevent my being the worst caretaker on earth. I would give him his meds, change his diaper with my eyes closed, then lock myself in the bathroom and weep. Sometimes, I heard him call for me, but I stayed in the bathroom, reading. I lived on Jelly Belly jelly beans and tortilla chips. I lost his dachshund.* One hot afternoon I thought my dad was already dead. I immediately called his hospice nurse to come pronounce it. He had told me the first thing I should do after he passed was to take the gold braided ring he wore on his little finger, which had belonged to his mother, and her mother before that. A true family heirloom. I was sweating, shaking, and weeping as I tried to wrench it off

---

* Woodrow was found later inside the pantry, perched on a mound of kibble inside a forty-pound bag of dog food, chowing down. At least *he* was being his best dog self.

his finger. The commotion woke him up. He hollered, "What in the hell is going on?"

Not my finest hour. And yet, my True Self at her best. I did what I thought I had to do, even if I did it inexpertly and with fear and trembling. I was neither poised, nor thinking happy thoughts. I was a wreck of greasy hair, a zitty chin, and coffee-stained sweatpants. I was so disastrously imperfect in that moment, and yet when my father finally did die, and I was able to remove his ring and slip it on my own finger, I felt I had done my best. There were no wouldas, couldas, shouldas. I was simply sad.

A thought experiment: what would your life look like if you were somehow able to arrive at the ever-receding mirage of the Ideal Female? Ta-da! Your body is now the perfect size and shape—not for you, but as judged by others. Your habits are impeccable. You have successfully embraced everything you've wanted to successfully embrace. You are productive, organized, and have mastered positive visualization. Now that you are your best self, what happens? Do you land the job or partner of your dreams? Are you promoted or proposed to? Do people love you more? Are parades held in your honor?

There is a catch: you must bid farewell to True Self. Everything you know to be true about who you are, all the imperfect, average, and less-than-culturally-approved habits, thoughts, and behaviors, is no more. True You, who you've suspected is holding you back from being Best You, has left the building.

Sit with this a bit. What would your life look like? Is it better?

Is it more interesting? Is the trade-off worth it? Is all the work to maintain best self—and there is a lot of it—something you're willing to do long term?

When I spent a day thinking about this, I was surprised to find I felt tender toward True Self, even though for most of my life I'd cursed her for getting in the way of my becoming the sort of perfect female I thought I was supposed to be. I thought again about best self being like an imaginary boyfriend and realized another reason people build relationships with imaginary beloveds—it's a way of having a loving relationship with yourself. Maybe, as Lizzo says, to become acquainted and make peace with our highly imperfect True Selves we need to be our own soul mates.

CHAPTER 5

A Short History of Self-Improvement During the Late Modern Age

Taught from their infancy that beauty is a woman's scepter, the mind shapes itself to the body, and, roaming round its gilt cage, only seeks to adorn its prison.
—Mary Wollstonecraft, *A Vindication of the Rights of Woman*

After my father died in 2000, I found a safety deposit box in the back of his closet. It was apparently the Very Important Document Repository. Inside, carefully folded, were the original family certificates—birth, marriage, death—a copy of the name change document—we were originally Karbowskis—and a tiny, tobacco-colored newspaper clipping from the *Detroit News* announcing that my mother was changing her name. In 1955, these announcements were common in newspapers. They appeared at the back, usually among the classified ads. The object of these little announcements was to enter the change into public record, thus proving you weren't a conman who went from town to town changing your name when it suited you. My mother had obtained a court order to change her name from Joan Mary Rex to Joan Mary Sharkey.

This was the first time I'd ever heard the name Rex. The Sharkeys were my mother's people, and that funny name (sharks!) was one of the few things I knew about them. Sometime in the early part of the twentieth century George and Maude Sharkey emigrated from Ireland and settled in Ypsilanti, Michigan. Maude ran a boarding house and had three daughters, Lorraine and Julia, two years apart, and then twenty years later, my mother. I must have been in second grade when I learned about the age gap. I asked my mother what the deal was; she laughed from behind the smoke of her cigarette and said she'd been "the child of old loins." Apparently, George had lived long enough to help conceive her, then was coming home drunk from the bar one night, was hit by a train, and died. By the time I was born George and Maude were long dead; Lorraine and Julia lived with their husbands in Detroit, and we lived in California and rarely saw them. That was the extent of what I knew about the Sharkeys.

The newspaper clipping was dated a scant four months before my parents married. Unlike Lorraine and Julia, who'd married assembly-line workers employed by the Ford Motor Company, my mother snagged my father, an industrial designer and engineer. Aha! I thought. My tidy, class-conscious suburban housewife mom must have been married to Mr. Rex before she married my dad, and didn't want that name forever immortalized on her marriage certificate. I immediately conjured up a short, passionate, disastrous marriage to a handsome ne'er-do-well like her father. A marriage of which she'd been profoundly ashamed and had kept secret.

I immediately called a friend who worked as a public investigator and told him about the ancient newspaper clipping and my suspicion that my mother had had a first marriage. Within forty-five minutes he called back. He'd easily managed to obtain two documents: my mother's birth certificate and her original request for the name change from the *Detroit News*, in which she revealed the reason for her request.

I'm going to stop right here. You're probably wondering what a crumbling sixty-five-year-old newspaper clipping has to do with swearing off self-improvement. How does something my mother did in the mid-twentieth century relate to figuring out how to live life as your True Self? My mother lived, and possibly died, before you were born. She's a stranger to you—and to me, it turned out.

Let us recall: to swear off spending a lifetime devoted to self-improvery it's necessary to be armed with the knowledge about how the world really works. The reality that everyone you imagine is judging you is *not* judging you, because they aren't even thinking about you, helps alleviate our shame. Wising up to the reality that the function of advertising is to stoke our insecurity, self-doubt, and self-loathing helps to loosen the grip of mass culture and rampant consumerism. Recognizing that the endless pursuit of self-improvement can make you feel crazy because it *is* completely fucking crazy, a Kafkaesque adventure where you should strive to be good, but not too good, because then you risk being unlikable, and there's nothing worse than being unlikeable, confirms that the game is rigged, and helps reinforce what I hope is a growing sense that there is a better way to live. Likewise, an understanding of history gives us even more room to contemplate the idiocy of most self-improvement schemes and regimes. It gives us a broader perspective, a practice that is so underutilized these days, to employ it on a regular basis is practically a superpower.

Furthermore, you don't want to be like Meghan McCain, do you? When she appeared on *Real Time with Bill Maher* in 2009, in her role as precocious political pundit and the GOP's new blonde to watch, she revealed herself to be the type of self-absorbed millennial who gives millennials a bad name. The topic of conversation was whether then president Obama was at fault for something or other, and one of the panelists referenced some crime or misdemeanor of the Reagan administration. McCain saucily admitted she knew nothing about the Reagan administration because "I wasn't born yet." After which she *giggled*. To which CNN political analyst Paul Begala said, "I wasn't born during the French Revolution, but I know about it."

Appreciating that history didn't begin the day you were born allows you to comprehend that regardless of your relationship with your mother, she too was trying to live up to some impossible female ideal. If, like Mary Wollstonecraft, she got the message that "beauty is a woman's scepter, the mind shapes itself to the body, and, roaming round its gilt cage, only seeks to adorn its prison," chances are she passed that "wisdom" on to you. If she was raised to believe that a woman should crush it at Harvard, build a brilliant career, and lean waaaaaay in, then she probably passed *that* wisdom on to you. Unless you're lucky enough to possess a female forebear who was a cheroot-smoking intellectual, bronc-busting cowgirl, sassy showgirl, or some other type of proto fuck-it-all outlaw, chances are the women who came before you felt considerable pressure to conform to their own standards of ideal womanhood.

What I learned about my own mother was this: that her real parents were not George and Maude Sharkey from Ypsilanti, Michigan, but a pair of teenagers who lived one town over. Her birth certificate revealed that they were Calvin Rex, nineteen, and Nora Kerrigan, seventeen. Their child, Joan Mary Rex, somehow came into the care of Maude Sharkey—evidence seems to point to my mother being left at the boarding house—who raised her but never formally adopted her. On the request to formally change her name, my mother wrote: "I would like to change my name to that of my foster mother, the only mother I have ever known."

Suddenly, so much made sense about my mother's anxiety that I would never find love, her endless concern that I might be cast out for being who I was. I tried to imagine how it must have been for her in the boarding house, the only child of Maude, after her older "sisters" had married and moved out. Was she afraid she might be sent away for failing to be cheerful and docile? Did she wonder why she was never formally adopted? All the people who have the answers are dead, so I'll never know. But I do know this: we are the daughters of women who spent their lives struggling to meet the impossible cultural demands of their time. Because of that, we should cut them some slack, which, in turn, will allow us to cut ourselves some slack.

The late modern period coincided with the Industrial Revolution and the rise of consumerism. This seems like a good place to begin our short history, for reasons that will make all too much sense in a moment. The Industrial Revolution began in Great Britain and spread to the United States in the late nineteenth century. Before that, most of the goods regular people needed were made at home. Cottage industries were literally industries in your cottage. People lived in villages or small towns, working the farm, minding the shop, crafting goods by hand. Women labored alongside the men and were recognized as an integral part of the household. They made soap, bread and butter, cloth and clothing, and medicine. It was *all* artisanal, handcrafted farm to table, bean to bar, barn to yarn, sheep to sweater. Every family was a self-supporting hub of industry and everyone pitched in. The family couldn't survive economically without women and their many skills.

Then new machine technologies were imported from England, and all the necessary goods—and a lot of unnecessary goods, as we shall see—began to be manufactured in factories. The goods made in factories were cheaper than the artisanal goods made in cottages, so the demand for cottage goods declined. Families left the farms for the mills, mines, and factories of more populous towns and cities. The public arena was born, and men were a part of it.

A small percentage of women were also employed by textile mills and coal mines. Because of their smaller size, they were often used to haul carts full of coal through the dark, narrow shafts, with a leather strap around their waist and a chain between their legs. For this, they were paid half as much as men. In a classic double-bind moment, even though their smaller size made them indispensable, they were despised for sacrificing their female virtue, their only treasure, by going to work in the first place.

Wages were low, hours long, conditions horrendous; in the early twentieth century a progressive political movement fought for and won better pay, fewer hours, and safety measures that transformed work from a place where you might lose a limb before lunch to much-relied-upon employment. There were no benefits, other than a paycheck.

Nevertheless, a middle class comprising merchants, businessmen, and bureaucrats began to emerge. One marker of the middle class was that they bought stuff they didn't need, fancy stuff that made them seem more on par with the wealthy aristocratic class, to distinguish them from the unskilled laborers beneath them. Another marker was a stay-at-home wife. She was the original trophy wife, whose leisure telegraphed her husband's success.

At the end of the nineteenth century, the Woman Question, which had been tossed around for five hundred years or so, gained fresh urgency. Translated from the French, *querelle des femmes*, the Question had doubts lurking beneath concerning the fitness of women to handle basic human rights. Women were viewed no differently than children, unable to reason, control their emotions, or hold a complex thought in their heads. Before the Victorian era, the Woman Question was mostly just a popular topic bantered around among philosophers and intellectuals who would get shit-faced in the local pub and blather about it till closing time. Should women be allowed to go out alone in public? Should they be permitted to express their opinions? Own property? Could women be trusted to do all the things men did—read, write, study, manage the household accounts—or was it the equivalent of leaving the family business to a hedgehog? English philosopher John Locke (1632–1704) argued that regardless of gender, the newborn human's mind is a blank slate, a tabula rasa. As we grow, we acquire both knowledge and prejudice; therefore women are no different from men in their abilities to successfully function in the world. A generation later French writer Jean-Jacques Rousseau (1712–1778) insisted that women by nature are subservient to men: "The man should be strong and active; the woman should be weak and passive. . . . When this principle is admitted, it follows that woman is specifically made for man's delight."

Inherent in the Question was a realpolitik component: what to *do* with this new class of women. As the nineteenth century surged into the twentieth, as factories and machines became more efficient, and as businesses became larger and more complex, the middle class continued to expand, and every woman who could afford to remain at home did so. A new, robust, and stratified bourgeois class blossomed, with capitalists and industrialists at the top; bankers, attorneys, academics in the middle; and blue-collar workers on the lowest rung. In the early part of the century, capitalists had joined the ranks of the upper class (much to the chagrin of the aristocrats), and the middle class expanded further. If you were a successful tradesman, you could now count yourself part of the petite bourgeoisie.

The middle-class wife went about shaping herself into a signifier of her family's affluence in the market economy. *Godey's Lady's Book*, published between 1830 and 1878, helped her figure out how to do this. It published articles on fashion, hygiene, health, and how to ride a horse sidesaddle. Each issue also published the sheet music for popular songs to be played on the pianoforte and the poems and stories of nineteenth-century literary greats Harriet Beecher Stowe, Edgar Allan Poe, and Nathaniel Hawthorne. *Godey's* was a source of inculcation, teaching women how to be refined within the domestic sphere, the only place they were fit to inhabit. And the more refined they were, the more they succeeded at femininity.

"The Angel in the House," the famously execrable poem by Coventry Patmore, outlined the perfect feminine personality, the one to which women should all aspire.[*] She should be graceful, gentle, submissive, self-sacrificing, uncomplaining, and sweetly dim. She existed to produce heirs and to soothe and flatter her husband.

"A successful man could have no better social ornament than an idle wife. Her delicacy, her culture, her childlike ignorance of the male world gave a man the 'class' which money alone could not buy," writes Barbara Ehrenreich and Deirdre English in *For Her Own Good: Two Centuries of the Experts' Advice to Women*. Women had to work very hard to improve themselves—to become less fully human and become more conventionally feminine.

The successful "The Angel in the House" brought to heel

---

[*] The poem was overlooked when it was published in England in 1854 but gained popularity in the United States at the end of the century. Further evidence that the United States falls far behind the rest of the developed world in its ability to tell a good poem from a bad one.

every "unpleasant" aspect of her personality. If she was smart, she played dumb or kept quiet; if she was logical, she feigned irrational emotionalism; if she was self-reliant, she pretended to be incompetent and needy; if she was confident, she learned to lower her eyes with a shy, self-deprecating smile.

Virginia Woolf, speaking before the National Society for Women's Service in 1931, had had enough of the insufferable, boring, martyr-y angel. When Woolf was invited to write a book review, normally a privilege reserved for male writers, she told how she had been forced to kill off the angel before she could proceed. "She [the Angel in the House] slipped behind me and whispered: 'My dear, you are a young woman. You are writing about a book that has been written by a man. Be sympathetic; be tender; flatter; deceive; use all the arts and wiles of our sex. Never let anybody guess that you have a mind of your own. Above all, be pure.'"

Meanwhile, less affluent women, then as now, still worked; they had no choice. The livelihood of their families depended on it. They still worked in factories and mills (the Mines and Collieries Act of 1842 forbade them from working underground). They worked in sweatshops. During World War I, they worked in bomb-making plants. They cleaned homes and offices. They waited tables in bars and diners. They were secretaries and typists. Like Maude Sharkey, the woman who I thought was my grandmother, they ran boarding houses. They were the living, breathing answer to the Woman Question—clearly women can get and keep their shit together enough to hold down a job and take care of their families at home—but nobody much was asking it about them. They labored in anonymity in part because they had little to contribute to the burgeoning consumer culture. They weren't free to buy things they didn't need, or that would communicate the wealth of their family or impress the neighbors.

The more cultured a woman was, the more leisure she enjoyed, the wealthier her husband was, the more she was liable to be sickly, by which I mean sick in a trendy way that indicated what a delicate flower she was. Illness became a marker of the upper-class wife. Neurasthenia was a popular ailment, a vague illness consisting of low energy, unexplained "nervous" headaches, and bad moods. A rich woman might easily spend her days feeling faint, suffering from nerves, and retiring to her room in the afternoon with a headache. The week of her menstrual period, the week before, and the week after, she rarely arose from her sickbed. She mastered the art of looking ethereal and ravishingly beautiful, while also appearing to be at death's door. If she was too hale and hearty, she might tuck into the arsenic. Then she was really sick. Imagine a sort of proto-heroin chic. Does this sound vaguely familiar? That to be truly feminine, in the eyes of the culture, you must be too weak to stand up? In my compulsive dieting days, I remember that feeling well.

Hysteria was another malady du jour exclusive to well-off women. No one quite knew what caused it; the early Greeks believed it was caused by the womb wandering around the body.

Symptoms included insomnia, anxiety, irritability, both sexual desire and lack of sexual desire, and "tendency to cause trouble for others." For a time, the cure was "pelvic massage," wherein the doctor would paddle her pink canoe until the patient was feeling relaxed and happy.

It was a status symbol for a rich man to send his wife to expensive health spas. Also, he would keep a small army of doctors on retainer, other men who would sweep in and minister to his wife, without ever curing her. To be a woman of a certain class meant to always have something undefinable wrong with you. If you squint, you can see the dim outline of modern self-improvement, where to be a desirable woman means always being in perpetual need of fixing.

A word about doctors. The medical industry as we know it was also in its infancy. The American Medical Association was formed in 1847, right around the time it started to become clear that to survive in the market economy, doctors needed patients, and a lot of them. How convenient, then, that apparently just being female was an incurable ailment.

Psychologist and educator G. Stanley Hall, writing in a 1905 treatise on the tortures of being female, quoted a Dr. Engelmann, the president of the American Gynecology Society and my personal favorite for winner of the Most Overwrought Extended Metaphor of the Twentieth Century Award: "Many a young life is battered and forever crippled in the breakers of puberty; if it cross these unharmed and is not dashed to pieces on the rock of childbirth, it may still ground on the ever-recurring shallows of menstruation, and, lastly, upon the final bar of the menopause ere protection is found in the unruffled waters of the harbor beyond the reach of sexual storms."

Medical "research" supported this seagoing conclusion. Women were tossed about by the mountainous ocean waves of completely normal lady biological business because it was believed we were ruled by the uterus. "It is as if the Almighty, in creating the female sex, had taken the uterus and built up a woman around it," proclaimed a professor M. L. Holbrook, in a speech to a medical society in 1870. Dr. G. L. Austin completely disagreed. *He* believed the ovaries reigned as maximum overlord of the female body, "giv[ing] woman all her characteristics of body and mind."

Every ailment was attributed to a woman's reproductive system, and thus demanded treatment. Got a sore throat? Must be related to some lady-bits malfunction. Too opinionated, too independent-minded, too interested in sex, or, conversely, not at all interested? Let's take a look at your vajayjay. Leeches placed on the vagina was a popular first step to curing whatever (sometimes they got lost in there). Various concoctions were injected into the uterus—water and milk, linseed oil, marshmallow infusion—and when that didn't work, cauterization of the cervix, often with no anesthetic save a nip of whiskey. As doctors became more adept at surgery that too became an option. By 1906, 150,000 women had had their ovaries removed.

I will pause to allow this to sink in.

In the same way that Botox and other spendy injectables are

the domain of the wealthy and well-off determined to "cure" aging today, these "treatments" were administered to upper- and upper-middle-class women, because they could afford them. And in any case, lower-class women, whose lives were harder by any measure, weren't particularly sickly. They got *sick*. Pneumonia, flu, and tuberculosis, lowbrow diseases, could kill them as well as anyone, but their overall robust health did nothing to dissuade the doctors from their beliefs; rather, it proved what the upper and middle classes had long suspected: that poor women were vulgar, coarse, and unrefined, more like oxen than the Angel in the House.

Side note: a handy test to see if you should spend your time chasing the latest self-improvement trend is whether people without much disposable income are doing it, or should be do- ing it. Smoking is a good example. That shit will kill you, rich or poor. Eating more vegetables? A head of broccoli is a better investment in your health than a bag of Funyuns. Paying a per- sonal nutrition and wellness coach to text you to make sure you're including enough antioxidant-rich superfoods in your açai bowl? Yeah, no, not happening.

At the turn of the twentieth century, the expansion of consumerism-as-lifestyle propelled women off their collec- tive fainting couches and into a new role. It was as good an answer to the Woman Question as any. What should we do with women? Convince them their life's mission was to pur- chase all the stuff factories were turning out by the megaton.

The market economy was booming, and to ensure continued growth, someone had to do it. Who better than women, who could be so easily conned into believing a bar of soap could land them a husband?[*]

At the same time, the work of Austrian neurologist Sigmund Freud was making its way across the Atlantic. The teachings of Freud set the record straight: it turned out female behavior was a matter of psychology and not gynecology. Oops! Doctors, ever reluctant to admit they were wrong, stopped insisting on treating these untreatable lady ailments and looked elsewhere for new clientele.

---

[*] In 1911, an ad campaign for Woodbury facial soap ran an ad featuring the tagline: "A skin you love to touch." In addition to the creepy, disembodied, *Silence of the Lambs*–ish phrasing, the illustration accompanying the ad shows a delicate blond beauty in a peach-and–pale green dress sitting in an armchair. Behind her, a handsome rogue in a black suit is kissing her neck, as she looks off into the distance with an expression that can only be described as deep resignation. Presumably she is a willing participant in this Woodbury soap–fueled seduction, but her inscrutable expression tells us she would rather be home doing the 1911 version of bingeing Netflix. At first glance the bodice, which exposes her flawless décolletage, appears strangely avant-garde. Random tufts of peach-and–pale green fabric sprout from the neckline. There is one daring off-the-shoulder sleeve—then, with a jolt, you realize that the handsome rogue is in the process of ripping off the dress. The Wikipedia entry on the History of Advertising declares this to be one of the first uses of "sexual contact" to sell a product; it was one of the most popular ad campaigns in history. The campaign was selling not soap, of course, but the power to control a man, to force him to lose control and ravish you. Which you then would pretend wasn't happening, because it was also an era when women weren't permitted to enjoy being ravished, even as they purchased products to inspire it.

The era of female invalidism as a way of life was over. The neurasthenic woman with her mysterious debilitating illnesses became as passé as power suits are today. The Woman Question did not go away. It never does. The only thing that changes is the answer, and in the early 1900s, the answer was homemaking, which—hallelujah!—requires purchasing a lot of stuff. Miraculously, middle-class women arose from their sickbeds, threw off their corsets, stripped the bed, washed the sheets, and took a feather duster to the place. There were still underpaid servants to do the bulk of the work, but there was a new role for wives in the domestic sphere: they would herewith devote themselves to the myriad tasks of keeping a house clean, organized, well-run, and did I mention clean?

The new woman was a domestic scientist in her own right. Magazines, newspapers, and books encouraged her to work endlessly to improve both her cleaning technique and, more important for our discussion, *the way she thought about it*. She was expected not only to do the work but also to tame any wayward thoughts she may have had about it. Ellen Swallow Richards, the founder of home economics, wrote, "It is not a profound knowledge of any one or a dozen sciences which women need, so much as an attitude of mind which leads them to a suspension of judgment on new subjects, and to that interest in the present progress of science which *causes them to call in the help of the expert*, which impels them to ask, 'Can I do better than I am doing?' 'Is there any device which I might use?' 'Is my house right as to its sanitary arrangements?' 'Is my food the best possible?' 'Have I chosen the right colors and the best materials for clothing?' 'Am I making the best use of my time?'"

The italics are mine, as is the irritation that Ellen Swallow Richards believed her own gender was not up to the task of reading a booklet or magazine article and figuring out how to clean her own fucking house.* You, Ellen Swallow Richards, may have been the first woman admitted to MIT, where you studied chemistry—something that was made much of, I'm sure, that a *woman* could excel in science!—but that doesn't mean other women are so dim they must call in experts to judge them on their ability to mop the floor. This one-two punch should come as no surprise by now: create a scenario in which a woman must do something correctly, or else suggest she call in an expert, because without someone to "help" she will undoubtedly fail.

Around the same time, popular science embraced the new Germ Theory of Disease. Now, keeping house wasn't simply something for a woman to do, while also keeping her ensconced at home and away from the corrupting influences of the public arena; it was a matter of life and death. Her decisions over what cleaning products to purchase, the way she managed her family hygiene, and her self-discipline in the face of routine tasks that were insanely boring were no less important than

---

* Ultimately, I forgave her because she also invented the first sewage treatment plant. Think of life without that.

those of a general on the battlefield. Suddenly, the health of her family was at stake. Silent killers lurked. You could not pick up a woman's magazine from 1902 without reading an article about how germs were invading the home via library books, postage stamps, doorknobs, and baby bottles. A single mote of dust contained over three thousand germs.* Not only that, if you left your (sparkling-clean) windows open, germs might float on over from the tenements on the other side of town and infect your entire family.

Women needed to up their game so they didn't kill everyone in the house. For then and now, it was presumed we were never doing it right. There was always a better method, a more expensive cleanser, a better way to manage our household priorities, a way to improve. By 1920, high schools and colleges were offering home economics courses. In 1929, a household efficiency expert named Christine Frederick wrote a book called *Selling Mrs. Consumer*, a nearly four-hundred-page advice book aimed at advertisers, advising them how they could manipulate the fears and anxieties of the average homemaker.†

Everything that is once new gets old. World War I came and went. Just as female invalidism had gone out of style, so did the notion that keeping a clean house was a higher, holy calling. Housework itself didn't go away—the fetishizing of it had

---

* True. The fungi and bacteria in a single mote of dust cohabit with all of us. Aside from provoking allergies, our household microbes are largely friendly.

† Thanks, sister. For fuck's sake.

only created more chores—but women began to see it for what it was: no more interesting than what the servants used to do. They still did it—of course they did—and so do we.

Before the baby boomers arrived, no one thought much about children. They dropped out of your vagina, and after they got themselves together (walking, talking, able to button their trousers) they went to work, helped on the farm, or cared for the ones who came after them. During the Industrial Revolution, kids shared the same advantage as women; their small size made their presence in factories and coal mines a boon because they could squeeze into nooks and crannies. The economic realities of the Great Depression caused people to rethink this. Adults needed whatever work they could get. Those nooks and crannies suddenly didn't seem so small after all.

In 1938, after a federal law was passed prohibiting child labor in factories, kids were—how shall I put this—underfoot. I'm guessing it was around this time that men discovered what women had always known, that children were lovable, maddening, entertaining, and downright adorable. They were more than tiny contributors to the family economy, it turned out: they were actual human beings with their own personalities. Children also had their own *needs*, different from those of an adult, and those needs could only be met by their mothers. Young people began to enjoy what seemed to be a very long childhood, during which their mothers were expected to scurry around tending to them, just as they did their husbands.

In 1946 Dr. Benjamin Spock published a volume that would become one of the bestselling books in history: *The Common Sense Book of Baby and Child Care*. The message to mothers was refreshing and empowering: "You know more than you think you do." Dr. Spock was the first pediatrician to study the psychology of children and to encourage their parents to treat them as individuals. The book was huge, selling fifty million copies at the time of Dr. Spock's death in 1998.

Spock proposed two radical notions: that maternal instinct was innate, and that women had the common sense to follow it. Spock further believed that in mothering your baby, the best course of action was to be yourself. Motherhood, once just a part of life, became a woman's highest calling. She, and she alone, was tasked with raising the new generation. Notice, please, the flip side: it also saddles mom with all the work, and all the responsibility when something goes wrong.

Let's hit pause for a moment. You may see where this is going.

A pattern began to emerge. As the decades rolled past, the answer to the Woman Question changed in response to the needs of capitalism and the market economy. Women were tossed a bone, something that they were told only *they* could do—clean the house, manage the household, take care of the kids, etc. They were allowed to go about their menial business undisturbed until some new earthshaking theory came along. Public intellectuals, op-ed writers, marketers, and advertisers would stir the pot. The mass media, including women's magazines, did their part by contributing incendiary headlines. This would cause men to sit up and take notice; on second thought, maybe this woman-only occupation was far too important to be left in the hands of women, giving rise to a new class of experts (usually men, except gender traitor Ellen Swallow Richards, mentioned above) who scooped up money, prestige, and power writing books and giving seminars and lectures and in general holding forth, telling women how to improve the thing they'd been doing just fine all along.

As Dr. Spock's fame grew, and as the children he helped raise began to come of age, other experts started to wring their hands. A woman may be brimming with maternal instinct, but could it really be trusted? More to the point, could a mere woman, with her sketchy "instinct," really be trusted to raise *men*? I think you know the answer.

Around the same time Spock was remaking American parenting, Austrian psychologist René Spitz began studying the effect of material deprivation on infants. He came to the conclusion that every mental disorder in an adult could be directly traced to a corresponding disorder in the mother. A baby whose mother deprived him of appropriate and continuous emotional connection would become depressed. A baby whose mother alternately pampered him and treated him with "hostility" would be a son prone to hypermotility, also known as rhythmic rocking. (I am not making this up.) A decade or so later, Harvard Medical School professor Joseph Rheingold decided the news was even worse, that all mothers were one step away from tossing their babies off a bridge. He posited that every woman subconsciously wanted to kill her child, because in giving birth to a baby, she could no longer live in denial of the greatest tragedy of her life, being born female. His theory, developed during a dozen years of clinical experience and so-called inductive inference, resulted in the publication of *The Fear of Being a Woman: A Theory of Maternal Destructiveness* in 1964.* Clearly mothering was far too serious an occupation to be left to mothers. Spock had liberated them, but that liberation could be disastrous! Mothers could be overpermissive, but also too strict. They could be affectionate, but also cold and withholding. It turned out that there was more to a woman than dubious maternal instinct. There was an entire, complex human being wearing that apron, making those cookies, folding that laundry, soothing that fever; could that human being be trusted? Answer: no. Every year nine gazillion parenting books are published. There are also apps—you knew there would be—including one to remind you your baby is in the car with you.

Not every girl went straight from her father's house to her husband's. Young women from the upper classes, and often the daughters of progressive or intellectual fathers, went to college. Betty Goldstein attended Smith in 1938. She won a scholarship for her top grades and edited the school newspaper. After

---

* Rheingold's nutty notion was not widely accepted; still, it did nothing to damage his career.

she graduated summa cum laude in 1942, Goldstein received a graduate fellowship to study at Berkeley. She was an avowed leftist, articulate, and mouthy. She left academia to write for labor union publications, and it was while working for the United Electrical Workers' *UE News* that she met and married Carl Friedan, with whom she would have three children. While pregnant with their second, Betty Friedan was fired, and returned home to take care of the house and raise their kids. She continued to freelance from home.

Friedan surveyed her fellow Smithies for their fifteen-year reunion, and was dismayed, though probably not surprised, to find a universal sense of dissatisfaction among the women. Had they really gone to college to make beds, vacuum, scrub toilets, and burn pork chops? Was comparison shopping for laundry detergent really going to be the best use of their educations?

In 1963, she published *The Feminine Mystique*, an investigation into why housewives were tired and miserable. The Problem That Had No Name did have a name, of course. The boredom felt by upper- and upper-middle-class housewives was perhaps one of the original first-world problems. But that realization doesn't solve the issue. Nor does feeling guilty because you don't feel grateful for a roof over your head and a pan of lasagna in the fridge. This sense of being limited and labeled, of being battered by hundreds—no, thousands—of articles, essays, books, speeches, advertisements in magazines and newspapers, and television and radio commercials instructing you how to improve upon tasks you could already do with your eyes closed, was yet another iteration of Wollstonecraft's gilt cage.

The Feminine Mystique doesn't really hold up. The introduction is bracing, and some of Friedan's riffs could and should be transformed into a rap by Missy Elliott: "A baked potato is not as big as the world, and vacuuming the living room floor—with or without makeup—is not work that takes enough thought or energy to challenge any woman's full capacity." Then you get to chapter 12, where she compares being a suburban housewife to living in a comfortable concentration camp, and the whole thing goes off the rails.*

Even so, the book sold over a million copies; it was the best-selling nonfiction book of 1964. It's hard to say how many read it to the end, but no matter. It was the right message for the right time. Women were getting restive. Advertising, mass media, and popular culture had overplayed their hand. A 1960s ad for Dormeyer appliances features a row of small appliances, including an "automatic toaster." The copy reads: "WIVES. Look this ad over carefully. Circle the items you want for Christmas. Show it to your husband. If he does not go to the store immediately, cry a little. Not a lot. Just a little. He'll go, he'll go. Husbands: Look this ad over carefully. Pick out what your wife wants. Go buy it. Before she starts to cry."

---

* In her memoir, *Life So Far*, Friedan apologized, sort of: "But then I got carried away, and wrote the one chapter in *The Feminine Mystique* I now regret, 'The Comfortable Concentration Camp.'"

Let us return to women who worked, or "worked outside the home," as we've been trained to say. In the early sixties, not all women were safely tucked into their split levels, grinding their teeth while dusting the end tables. In 1960, 31 percent of all married women and 80 percent of all single women worked. That's a lot of women who didn't live perfect lives as portrayed on television and in the media, a lot of women for whom reality was not wall-to-wall carpets in the suburbs but a sack lunch in the steno pool.

Helen Gurley was one of these girls. Born in Arkansas in 1922, Gurley had none of the advantages of Betty Friedan's Smithie classmates. Her father died when she was ten, and her mother dragged Helen and her sister to Los Angeles, rather than allow neighbors to witness their descent into poverty. Helen was smart, and a hard worker, but she couldn't afford college and enrolled in secretarial school. For the next eighteen years she worked as a secretary, then as a copywriter. Think Peggy Olson, who was Gurley-esque with her smarts, ambition, and average looks.

Sex and the Single Girl, published after Helen Gurley married David Brown in 1959 at the age of thirty-seven, was the culmination of everything she knew about life as a woman on her own. "I think a single woman's biggest problem is coping with the people who are trying to marry her off," she wrote. She felt marriage was for when you were old, that in your twenties and thirties you should make the most of your youth by working hard and maybe having a nice affair with the boss. She was a cheerful can-do radical with a hair-sprayed flip and an A-line dress. She thought wives were boring, and she thought husbands thought their wives were boring. "The sexiest women are the achievers, for they are the most interesting and exciting. They challenge a man by being as desirable, sought after, and respected as he is."

It was the nonfiction hit of 1962, selling two million copies in three weeks, and eventually lead to HGB's reign at *Cosmopolitan*, where she ruled as editor in chief for thirty-two years. Gurley's readership was average young women like herself, "mouseburgers" who came from nowhere and nothing but yearned for a life of romance and glamour. Her bosses thought she was crazy—how many single women who thought there was a satisfying life to be lived away from husband, home, and hearth could there be? Millions, it turned out. *Cosmopolitan* was and still is the bestselling women's magazine in the world.

By 1973 women were given the right to choose, and in 1974 they were permitted to open credit accounts without a male cosigner. Feminism was *on*. Women left their husbands in record numbers, and attended consciousness-raising groups where they gazed at their vaginas with a hand mirror. They had had enough. They were giddy, thumbing their nose at all the female stereotypes and imperatives that came before. They had birth control; they had access to abortion. It was revealed that the world was groaning with humans, so if you chose to have one child or no children at all, you were doing everyone a favor.

Then, in the blink of an eye (okay, a decade or so), Helen Gurley Brown went from sex-positive trailblazer to embarrassment. Second-wave feminists accused her of being a retro man-pleaser. Nora Ephron wrote, on the endless health of *Cosmopolitan*'s sales numbers, "She is demonstrating, rather forcefully, that there are well over a million American women who are willing to spend sixty cents to read not about politics, not about the female-liberation movement, not about the war in Vietnam, but merely about how to get a man." Ephron was not wrong. We do want to know how to get a man, or a woman. We want love, even when it's politically unfashionable.

In the mid-1970s women had more freedom than ever, but while everyone was busy making up for lost time, clubbing in platform shoes and doing coke off the mirrors of strange men with feathered hair and flowered Qiana shirts (we've moved on to the disco era), the old expectations weren't hauled off to the cultural junkyard, where they eventually disintegrated and blew away. Instead the expectations society and culture had of women, and women had of themselves, grew.

No matter how many clubs they closed or strangers they went home with, most women were still expected to get married. Once she became a wife and mother, it was the same old same old. Wives were still expected to keep a clean, well-run, germ-free home. Mothers were still expected to raise the children and, increasingly, to enrich their lives. The laundry wasn't going to fold itself, and someone had to put dinner on the table. Which remains true right this minute.

Feminism + more women enrolling in college + more women launching careers before marriage = more women in the workforce than ever before. By 1980, half of America's women worked, regardless of marital status. From 1972 to 1985, the number of women entering "management" jobs nearly doubled, growing from 20 to 36 percent. By 1985 half of all college graduates were women, and they were making their way into professional careers.

While women were making inroads into the workplace, they were reminded that the smarter and more successful they were, the less likely they were to get married. The famous 1986 *Newsweek* cover fake-worried on our behalf about "The Marriage Crunch." A graph beside the headline, "If you're a single woman, here are your chances of getting married," delivered the bad and erroneous news. (In fact, women with college degrees are more likely to get married and stay married than women without.)

Up until this moment in history, most people didn't feel entitled to have everything they wanted. There were only twenty-four hours in a day, a person couldn't be in two places at once, and you could only give 100 percent of your attention and best efforts to that which mattered most. A man couldn't be a playboy on the Riviera while also working hard enough to make partner at a law firm. He couldn't be a rodeo clown while also managing hedge funds on Wall Street. He couldn't sail the high seas while also working ninety-plus hours as a trauma surgeon at an inner-city ER.

But you know what all men could have?

A career, a wife, and kids. Plus, a weekly poker game or standing golf date.

Could women who worked as hard as men at their careers have the same thing? It was 1982, and the debate barely got off the ground before Helen Gurley Brown, still arguably the most powerful woman in media, published *Having It All: Love, Success, Sex, Money, Even If You're Starting with Nothing.* Once "having it all" hit the cultural bloodstream, we became convinced that, yes, we could have it all. We could have everything we want. Having it all became code for having a soaring professional career, a happy and hot marriage, cool, well-adjusted kiddos, and, of course, looking thin and fit and fuckable. If you didn't have it all, or want it all, you were deficient.

For a decade or so, we were made to believe we could have it all if we worked from predawn to postdusk, got superorganized, and were able to enlist our husband to help out around the house. I gave birth to my daughter in 1992, and that was the game plan. Her father and I agreed we would have only one child, because we knew we both wanted to work full-time. We split the day care and the housework the best we could. The marriage failed for other reasons, but for a few years, I had it all.

Twenty-eight years later, having it all is as divisive and triggering as ever. In a famous 2012 cover story for the *Atlantic*, former State Department director of policy planning Anne-Marie Slaughter called it out for the ridiculous, unachievable bullshit it is. In her 2018 memoir, *Becoming*, former first lady Michelle Obama wrote, "Marriage still ain't equal, y'all. It ain't equal. I tell women that whole 'you can have it all'—mmm, nope. Not at the same time. That's a lie. It's not always enough to lean in, because that [expletive] doesn't work."

For what it's worth, *Having It All* was not Helen Gurley Brown's original title. According to her biographer, Jennifer Scanlon, in an interview with the *New York Times*, Gurley Brown wanted to call her book *The Mouseburger Plan.** She had envisioned her book for "the downtrodden" woman, and she felt *Having It All* made her sound like "a smart-ass-all-the-time winner." She and her husband, David Brown, had no children themselves, yet having it all would become shorthand for everything to which women in the twenty-first century should aspire. The title *Having It All* was the idea of the marketing department, and then as now, the marketing department always wins.

There's a House that Jack Built quality to the expectations surrounding women in the late modern era: this is the woman who pulls down six figures, who manages the house, who raises the

---

* A terrible title. It sounds like a diet where you only eat burgers made of mice.

kids, who supports the husband, who makes the bone broth and juices the carrots, who runs the half marathons, who whitens her teeth, who rocks the bikini well into perimenopause, who lives in the house built by mass marketing, media, and advertising.

The second shift was identified by sociologist Arlie Russell Hochschild in her 1989 bestseller of the same name. It identified all the sack lunch–making, laundry-doing, meal-planning, living room–tidying, and toilet paper roll–replacing women did in addition to holding down a full-time job in the so-called formal workforce. It's the work women do on top of the work that women do. Men help more than they used to, but it's still by and large on us. The third shift, coined by Naomi Wolf in 1992, is all the "appearance work" we're required to do in addition to everything else. By now you know the drill: while giving 110 percent at work, showing up for every T-ball practice with the correct snacks, cooking healthy meals, and doing more than our share when it comes to scrubbing the toilets and picking up everyone's dirty socks, we must also have silky hair, flawless skin, bee-stung lips, a sassy pedicure, and tank top–worthy triceps, and be able to rock a miniskirt at a moment's notice.

I'm going to suggest a fourth shift, where we must do all of the above, with a flawless parade of positive thoughts and vigorous affirmations. The fourth shift encompasses all the work we're supposed to be doing on our inner selves as well. Take a spin through the latest offerings on Medium, and you'll see what I mean. A sample: "21 Behaviors That Will Make You

Brilliant at Creativity and Relationships." "10 Mental Hacks to Start and Finish What You Hate." "How to Be the Type of Person Everyone Wants to Know."

Now, thanks to the fourth shift, we've got to be exercising and toning our inner selves as well. Neuroplasticity is all the rage these days. The brain can be trained as easily as a treat-motivated spaniel, it turns out. And since it *can* be trained, it *should* be. Reading is no longer something you do for fun, but to build empathy. Keeping a journal is no longer something else you do just because you enjoy keeping a record of your days and are a little in love with your own handwriting, but "a powerfully transformative keystone habit."[*] Going for a walk is no longer a thing you do when you need to stretch your legs and get the dog to stop staring at you; it's a way to increase the size of your hippocampus. Which, aside from our breasts, is the only other part of our body that is allowed to be large.

In 2020, the cultural mandate for women is a version of Nike's iconic imperative. Just Keep Improving. Life is an ongoing, down-to-the-studs remodel. Self-improvement has become a way of life.

---

[*] Listen, I've kept a journal since I was ten, and I can tell you it's just one long rant about people who are pissing me off.

PART II

CHAPTER 6

Where the Wild Things Still Are

Let everything happen to you: beauty and terror.
Just keep going. No feeling is final.

—Rainer Maria Rilke

Prior to the 2008 housing crash, when you could literally wish for a subprime mortgage and some shady broker would make it so, Rhonda Byrne's 2006 *The Secret* burst onto the self-improvery scene. It has sold roughly a zillion copies and was translated into every language on earth. Oprah and many of your favorite influencers endorse it, while Mark Manson, the King of Fuckistan himself, wrote, "*The Secret* teaches self-absorption and blind acceptance of your emotions, and I call bullshit on all of it."

I believe in giving things a try before calling bullshit, and

I feel I've given manifesting a fair shake. I'll just say this: it's all well and good to act as if you've already sold the house and landed the job, but don't make financial decisions based on something that hasn't happened.* Live and learn. And what I learned is that the Universe cannot be conned. It has taken my measure and finds me far too fond of bitching and moaning and other displays of negativity to grant me my wishes.

I have mixed feelings about doing affirmations. The science behind it is sound, or at least it doesn't depend on attributing consciousness to an inconceivably vast cosmic vacuum inhospitable to all human life except on this crumb of dust we call home. Research reported in the November 2015 issue of *Social Cognitive and Affective Neuroscience* found that self-affirmations do affect our well-being, reducing stress and giving us a better outlook on life in general. Consider one of my preferred affirmations: "I am at peace with who I am." My conscious mind might disagree, especially if I'm in a department store with its usual cruel dressing-room lighting trying on a bathing suit, but my brain buys it. The stimulation in my medial prefrontal cortex and posterior cingulate cortex, the parts of the brain where most of our self-related processing occurs, is the same, regardless of whether the affirmation is true.

---

* Thanks for the loan, Ann, Connie, Scott, Ed, and any other friends who've lent me money and whose names I've forgotten. Pay you back as soon as I can manifest some cash.

Even patently untrue affirmations can be beneficial. If you're due to give a big presentation at work and you walk into the conference room thinking, "I'm the smartest person in the room," the affirmation doesn't magically make it so. In that we can agree on what constitutes intelligence, you're probably not the smartest person in the room. Maybe you are, whatever. The point is, affirming this to yourself will make you behave in a way that's more confident and assertive, increasing the likelihood that your presentation will go better. You'll feel better and more confident, your boss will be thrilled you didn't blow it, and after work drinks are on her.

That said, I'm a situational affirmationist. Telling yourself, "This is perfectly safe and I'm going to have the time of my life" as you're standing at the open door of an airplane with your parachute on is one thing; feeling obligated to chant a dozen affirmations before you get out of bed in the morning only builds a habit of self-distrust. We start to feel we can't just get on with it without telling ourselves it will all be okay. Furthermore, too many affirmations uttered too often under too many circumstances tend to reinforce our feeling that we need to do something to fix ourselves, and you know how I feel about that.

I recommend a balanced diet of affirmations, critical thinking, and common sense, seasoned with skepticism and black humor. Of course, this flies in the face of the orthodoxy of self-improvement, which demands our minds be as smooth and exfoliated as our foreheads, free of all thoughts that are troubling or ambivalent. Every day in every way, we scrupulously make sure our thoughts are positive, that we're never disapproving or judgmental. We reassure people we don't know on Facebook that things will work out, that they've got this. We send them light and love. I'm the first one to respond to something witty or well-observed with "I love you!" It's oppressive, this unspoken pressure to be of good cheer every goddamn day.

The recent exception to the happy thoughts-a-thon at the center of most self-improvement projects is anger. The cauldron of female fury hath finally bubbled over, and it's about fucking time. The late twenty-teens witnessed an onslaught of books, articles, and political moments supporting the expression of female rage. In 2013 #BlackLivesMatter was founded by Alicia Garza, Patrisse Cullors, and Opal Tometi, after George Zimmerman's acquittal in the death of Trayvon Martin. In 2006 civil rights activist Tarana Burke adopted the hashtag #MeToo to bring attention to the ubiquity of sexual abuse in women's lives; in 2017 actress Alyssa Milano reinvigorated the discussion after the explosion of allegations of abuse by Harvey Weinstein, imploring every woman who's ever been sexually assaulted to share her #MeToo story, and her rage. In 2018 three big books celebrating the power of women embracing their anger hit the shelves: *Eloquent Rage: A Black Feminist Discovers Her Superpower* by Brittney Cooper (February); *Rage Becomes Her: The*

Power of Women's Anger by Soraya Chemaly (September); and *Good and Mad: The Revolutionary Power of Women's Anger* by Rebecca Traister (October).

These books were roundly celebrated, garnering good reviews and landing on many best book of the year lists. As well they should. As a woman who is always slightly pissed off at something or other, I welcomed their publications, bought them in hardcover, gave them away to friends, and bought them *again* in hardcover. These books take no prisoners, but a Bustle review summed up my feeling that something was not quite right—not with the books, but with their reception.

> *Eloquent Rage* shows readers the many ways anger can be an effective tool—or, as Cooper puts it, a superpower—in the fight for change. . . .
>
> *Rage Becomes Her* makes a case [that] . . . expressing anger isn't only important for individual well-being, but crucial for enacting serious societal change. . . .
>
> *Good and Mad* is an insightful, inspiring, and razor-sharp look at just how important collective female anger has been and is in enacting change and impacting culture, politics, and the world.

This coming from you, Bustle? The subtextual notion is that anger and its expression are not simply a part of the normal human psyche, "important for individual well-being," but are only allowed and encouraged when necessary for the greater good. What if a woman is angry only on her own behalf? There are, after all, many kinds of anger. As Lilly Dancyger, editor of *Burn It Down: Women Writing About Anger*, writes in the introduction, "Our anger doesn't have to be useful to deserve a voice."

For what it's worth, another book on female anger was published in 2018, and is outselling the rest on Amazon by a substantial margin: Julie Catalano's *Anger Management Workbook for Women: A 5-Step Guide to Managing Your Emotions and Breaking the Cycle of Anger* (June). Proof, as though it's needed, that even though female rage is having a moment, most women aren't so sure they want it hanging around causing trouble.

Acknowledging the breadth and depth of our anger doesn't move us closer to perfection, or the feminine ideal, but it does make us whole. This is true whether you march in the street or spend an hour hitting tennis balls against the garage door or swimming laps in the pool, my teenage go-to moves when my mother would say, "You need to do something with that anger." Notice, please, she didn't say I shouldn't feel it. As mistaken as she was about so many things, my mother knew that anger needed to be addressed, not denied.

Which brings us to Carl Jung—a phrase that probably hasn't been uttered in many decades. A Swiss psychoanalyst, student of Sigmund Freud, and, along with Alfred Adler, founder of modern analytical psychology, Jung was popular among hippie pundits in the 1970s, or at least my friend Patty's older brother, Mike, who gave me a copy of *The Portable Jung* at an impressionable age. Mike was our weed dealer and taught philosophy at the local junior college, and I read the book straight through. I took to heart Jung's wisdom about learning to embrace my shadow side, a concept that was later confirmed by a therapist I saw for the better part of ten years. "Everyone carries a shadow," Jung wrote, "and the less it is embodied in the individual's conscious life, the blacker and denser it is."

To be human is to have a shadow, and the more we avoid it, deny it, or try to tamp it down, the more active, and potentially destructive, it becomes in our lives. The shadow is a crowded gathering, where our demons, evil twin, alter ego, and crazy unhinged bitch goddess party. Our so-called base animal urges are there too—the impulse to grab a burger out of a stranger's hand when you're hungry, fuck your best friend's husband behind the shrubbery at the neighborhood barbecue, or strangle the leader of your self-care book club. Why? Because you're a human being, and that's part of the show.

The shadow bulldozes right on through our twee affirmations. There is no healing your shadow side with positive thoughts. There is no convincing it to calm the fuck down with a cheery, upbeat mantra. "Every day, in every way, I'm getting better and better" means nothing to your shadow side. It is completely impervious to positive thinking.

How does this black, dense shadow show up in your life? It's a clever beast: what you can't accept in yourself, you can't accept in others. The shadowy aspects of yourself that you're afraid to acknowledge, you project onto other people.

The perfect dramatic representation can be found in Laura Dern's character, Amy Jellicoe, in HBO's short-lived dramedy *Enlightened*. After she has a full-on mascara-smeared-to-her-chin meltdown at work, Amy spends a couple months at a retreat in Hawaii. After she returns, she is "enlightened," but also as self-absorbed, manipulative, and enraged as she was before, even though she talks the right talk. The joke is not her New Age beliefs, but her complete lack of self-awareness and inability to accept her shadow side.

Internet callout and cancel culture exists because it feels much better to project your shadow onto other people, especially when you don't have to look them in the eye. I'm not talking about righteous expressions of anger in response to world events, social injustice, and you know the rest, but the finger-pointing, name-calling, insulting, and holier-than-thou judging, from the right, the left, and everyone in between—I'm assuming there are still some out there—directed at other people who've done nothing more than expressed a different opinion.

To further complicate matters, our shadow side includes qualities deemed unacceptable by society and our family. Often these traits revolve around gender. In earlier generations boys were trained not to show their feelings, while girls were trained not to show their competence and leadership abilities.

Or their anger, come to that. Your parents, teachers, other authority figures, and peers might have punished you, or not invited you to the slumber party, for exhibiting these traits as a little girl, and thus you hid them, stuffing your ambition, your will, your strength, and your desires to make your way in the world on your own and to state your opinions with no apologies in the back of some far-off storage unit of the mind. Millennials are smarter on this front, and presumably twenty-first-century parents will avoid shaming their children for failing to exhibit the proper gendered behavior, although they've got the Battle of the Almighty Screen to wage. I don't envy them.

Do women have deeper, denser shadows than men? I'm guessing yes. Remember the Angel in the House? That bitch has become the Guest Who Wouldn't Leave. We still somehow feel the need to suppress qualities that might be viewed as positive were they exhibited by men, because power, strength, ambition, aggression, anger, and speaking your mind with passion and clarity, otherwise known as being "shrill," are still considered negative female traits.

This brings us back to feelings of shame, the source of much of our drive to improve ourselves. Recall the definition: ". . . the intensely painful feeling or experience of believing we are flawed and therefore unworthy of acceptance and belonging." Our perceived flaws are often related to our shadow side. We've tucked so much of what we've been taught were unacceptable traits into our shadow that it takes very little to kindle shame, which is activated not when someone else is judging us, as it often seems, but when we are judging ourselves.

How do we cope with our negative self-assessment? We attempt to distance ourselves from it by staying silent and pretending it doesn't exist. We attempt to solve the shame through self-improvery. Or we try to "beat" shame by projecting it onto others.

This is evident when you're being an asshole for no discernable reason.

Like most women, I wasn't an innocent bystander in the mommy wars. I've supported myself and often the whole family with my writing, which, as I've noted elsewhere, is like having a lemonade stand for a living. I chose this life. I enjoy this life. It's always interesting, if fiscally harrowing. That said, three weeks after my daughter was born, I had a huge deadline. My husband was a film sound designer and was out of town on a job. It was a dumb assignment that didn't even pay particularly well, and anyone else would have turned it down, by whom I mean anyone who wasn't desperate for money. Fortunately, I was a champion breastfeeder and my daughter was a champion breastfeedee. I hooked her up to one boob, freeing me to type with one hand. The day before the piece was due, I came down with a raging case of mastitis.

My new-mom friend Julia worked for a company in Portland that offered a very generous maternity leave package. The week before her maternity leave was up, she decided to quit to stay home with her son because her husband was in finance and made a boatload. When I told her about the dumb deadline and the mastitis—I still remember my teeth chattering with the fever/chill combo as I talked to her on the phone—she offered to come over to help with the baby so I could finish the piece. She had thoughtfully taken her son to her mother's house, so she could focus on taking care of my daughter. She brought some homemade pumpkin bread with her, which was very nice, and also as annoying as fuck.

She cut us each a slice of pumpkin bread and asked, "So how on earth did this happen?"

At that moment, I decided we could never be friends. She had an infant and the time to bake homemade pumpkin bread, while her husband was at work making money with other people's money, or whatever it is finance guys do. She wasn't one of those stay-at-home moms who came down with mastitis, because those who did, like me, were idiots who forgot that you needed to switch boobs, that you couldn't just hang your baby on your nipple the way you might hang a tote bag on a hook. I felt myself withdraw. The baby was napping anyway, and after we ate our bread I told her she didn't need to stick around. She looked perplexed. I never called her again, and when mutual friends wondered if I'd seen Julia lately, I said she was too bougie for me, and also, I couldn't stand how she thought she was all that—nineties speak for entitled. I knew what I was doing, having been an avid reader of *The Portable Jung*, but I did it anyway. I was pissed off at myself for pursuing two conflicting realities, and thinking because I desired them, I was entitled to them. I wanted to be a writer—I was a writer—but I spent money as if I were Julia, with her husband in finance. Had I accepted my choice, and budgeted accordingly, I wouldn't have needed to take the stupid assignment that led to my having to crash a deadline when my daughter was a newborn.

Jung believed it was a rare person who could ever truly confront his shadow. The best most of us can do is to identify our projections. To be aware that we're overreacting or casting harsh and often irrational judgment, for no reason that someone without our issues can see, is a small but important step toward inviting the shadow into consciousness. Leaving our shadow to molder like the leftovers at the back of the fridge, all the while chasing after the female ideal with her artificially generated happy thoughts, does nothing but deepen the darkness and keep us further alienated from our True Selves.

Self-policing our thoughts and feelings so that we're always reframing something unfortunate as a terrific opportunity, or telling ourselves that everything happens for a reason, or refusing to allow ourselves to accept traits that we've been led to believe have no place in our best self doesn't make us better people; it just makes us limited people.

We're so afraid of the messy stuff inside of us. In 1963, illustrator Maurice Sendak published a 338-word children's book that was panned upon publication and kept cropping up on banned-books lists. The pearl clutchers argued that *Where the Wild Things Are* was too dark and too negative for children. Sendak, born to Polish-Jewish immigrants in Brooklyn, knew all about the muck in the human soul. Most of his family had perished in the Holocaust. Given that, he thought kids were more complex and made of stronger stuff than people imagined.

The story is about a boy named Max whose mother sends him to bed without supper for misbehaving. To channel his rage, he enters a private jungle populated by fanged creatures over whom he reigns as king. Even though Max grows to love the wild things, and the wild things him, he decides to sail home to his room and to his family, whom he knew loved him. Waiting for him at home was his dinner, "still hot."

It remains one of the most beloved books of all time in part because of Sendak's message: we all have a wild thing inside of us, which we can manage with the help of our imagination. Rather than trying to improve the qualities that feel as if they don't jibe with what we imagine to be our best self, work with them. The ways in which we cope with the dark side, where the wild things are, is a component of our individuality. Remember the pumpkin bread Julia brought me that day? We found each other on Facebook a few years ago. She tried to recall the last time we'd seen each other—I remembered it exactly. When I mentioned the pumpkin bread, she LOLed. She said she'd baked it as a peace offering. I was momentarily confused. "Peace offering?" I typed.

"I was so jealous that you got to stay home with your baby *and* write, I had to do something. I felt like a total bitch!"

Just now this beautiful thought popped up on Instagram: "For every minute you are angry, you lose sixty seconds of happiness." Unless being angry makes you happy. Which would be one of those shadow-side things that one might be reluctant to admit to oneself. Speaking only for myself, I love a good, sweary, mean-spirited rant. And if that's part of your shadow side, you should too.

CHAPTER 7

True You Rising

I have accepted fear as part of life—specifically the fear of change . . . I have gone ahead despite the pounding in the heart that says: turn back. . . .

—Erica Jong

The first rule of yeah, no, not happening is come as you are. The person who says fuck it all is the person you are right this minute. There's no hopping in the wayback machine to undo the year you spent being bulimic or spending your paycheck on hair extensions, no throwing in the towel because you didn't take that scholarship or married that lunkhead straight out of high school. Our intention is not simply to stop doing the stuff we don't want to do, but also to dismiss the fantasy that if we were just *better*, our lives would be better. Part of this fantasy sometimes consists of, once again, imagining a down-to-the-studs remodeling of our personalities. Filled with resolve, we think, I'm saying no to all this bullshit, NOW!

Let's say you're someone who has put on makeup every morning for twenty years before you left the house. Or started a new diet every time you've felt a twinge of insecurity. Or worked extra hard to be nice to people you don't like, because you're afraid of coming off as a bitch. Or felt the need to crank up the holiday-making machine at the end of every year, for fear of neglecting your domestic duty. You're a woman who's been socialized in this culture, and some of this shit is ingrained, and the first thing to which we must all say yeah, no, not happening is further judging ourselves as flawed, inferior, imperfect.

In this moment, that's just you. Maybe you'll come to realize you can forgo the fake eyelashes, or whatever they're telling us we need this minute, maybe not. Is it a waste of time and money? For some yes, for others no. For some it's bowing to the impossible rules as set forth by the patriarchy, for others it's a way to have a few moments to collect yourself before the day begins and literally put on your game face. Maybe you'll come to realize you can safely dislike someone and still accord them the respect they deserve as a fellow human trying to make their way. Maybe you'll one day conclude that the holidays are a lot more fun when it's a group effort, and not, as my friend Connie says, "an annual festival put on by women for the enjoyment of men and children."

Even though I've said yeah, no, not happening to a lot of self-improvement, I have not sworn off many self-improvery habits that take time, money, energy, and may best be categorized as shoring up the ruins. I dye my hair. I have strong opinions about concealers. I am vain about my exquisite feet and I love sandals. Also purses and fine cotton T-shirts. I put on mascara before I go out of the house. Beneath the mascara I wear lash building primer even though I don't think it does any good. I've been known to get my eyebrows waxed. I don't get manicures, but I do have one of those buffer blocks that removes nail ridges. I have some forearm flab (yes, *forearm* flab) about which I despair but forget about until I see a picture of myself with my arms crossed. I exercise three or four times a week, but learned long ago to say yeah, no, not happening to any kind of athletic event that requires a training log. My eating regime involves staying away from potato chips, eating an apple a day, and having a green salad with dinner.

I have faith that if you're reading this book, you already have a good idea about the expectations from which you'd like to free yourself, and that's where you should start. The things you feel you "should" do but can't abide. The things that, when doing them, make you feel irritated or depressed. The things you believe to be a waste of time, energy, and money. The things that make you feel unknown to yourself.

I polled my friends, via email, over cocktails, and on social media, and here is a sample of when they're saying yeah, no, not happening, and the spirit in which they're saying it:

Yeah, No. Not Happening.

Any of those fucking "look at me" exercises (yeah, I'm talking to you, Zumba)

Being "not quite so overbearing"

Heels

Jogging

Choking down dietary supplements that, according to my doctor, result only in "very expensive pee"

Giving up carbs

Supporting middle-aged white guys in their misguided thinking

All bullshit pyramid schemes selling upscale skin care, supplements, and essential oils

Quinoa

Kale, kale, and did I mention kale?

Worrying about wrinkles

Blowing curly hair straight

Lipstick

Camping, hiking, and all that outdoorsy shit that's supposed to make you seem cool and adventuresome

Doing more than my share just to avoid a fight

Shapewear

Holding my tongue rather than calling people on their shit

Going to concerts, festivals, and parties where there's no seating

Opera

Bush-hair removal

The assumption that I am the "doer" in the house

Reiki nonsense

Motivational memes with the depth of a bumper sticker

Hiding my flabby upper arms

Clique-ish mom groups

Believing a clean house makes me a better woman

Pretending to be extroverted

Creepy self-help evangelists who tell you self-discovery costs $10,000 or a sustaining donation

Mommy wars

Phony-baloney positivity

Celery juice

Learning to speed read (why rush through something you enjoy, for fuck's sake?)

Being that woman who produces a Thanksgiving extravaganza, then trying to convince myself I'm grateful for the opportunity to spend hundreds of dollars on food and a week preparing a meal that is consumed in twelve minutes

Pretending to be excited over recipes, and cooking in general, when I'm just not, and also not feeling guilty or apologizing for this

Taking anything to the next level

A friend was in the women's locker room at the gym after a circuit-training class. She was a regular, as was the young woman using the locker next to hers. My friend said anyone would look at this young woman and find her fitter and prettier than most people. Out of the corner of her eye, my friend watched as the young woman squeezed herself into some shapewear, followed by a pair of jeans she had to jump up and down to zip. The young woman had literally broken a sweat. Then she put her feet, which had a Band-Aid on each heel, into a pair of stilettos. My friend and the woman traded glances, and my friend said, "That looks like an awful lot of work." The woman rolled her eyes and said, "I don't even know why I do it."

If you don't even know why you do it, try saying yeah, no, not happening, and see how that feels. If you find you still dig it, then carry on.

The afternoon of the morning I decided to swear off self-improvement I made a list of all the things I will never improve. It was exhilarating to say fuck it all to everything I felt I should be doing for reasons I couldn't even remember. After I made my list, I had a cup of coffee with whole milk and an old-fashioned doughnut. Then I had another doughnut, because I felt like it. I was relieved of guilt for skipping the greens in my morning smoothie, as I sometimes did, because I couldn't bring myself to face fucking Swiss chard at 8:00 a.m. Anyway, not that I was counting calories, because yeah, no, that was totally not happening anymore, but I bet my usual smoothies, made with berries, a frozen banana, some greens, protein powder, almond milk, almond butter, and a little honey, had as many calories—maybe more!—than two old-fashioned doughnuts. While I ate, I read William Finnegan's *Barbarian Days*, my favorite book of the decade, even though the few women who appear are underdeveloped girlfriends and wives, something I despised. I am aware that you're not supposed to eat and read at the same time, but yeah, no, not happening. The relief I felt was immense, as if I were on vacation from a very strict girls' academy that demanded perfection and did not grade on a curve.

It was 9:20 a.m. I hadn't journaled, tracked my productivity, exercised, meditated, rolled my eyes while I phoned in some affirmations (no wonder the universe wasn't cooperating), or planned the daily menu, making sure to include five (or was it nine now?) servings of fruits and vegetables, açai berries, and lots of turmeric. I loaded the dishwasher. I texted *Yoyo!* to my daughter—our way of checking in. I went out front and watered the begonias struggling to stay alive in the decorative pots on either side of the front steps. I went out back and picked up the dog poop. I deleted all my newsletter subscriptions to websites that peddled self-improvement, including the one I despised most, which conflates spirituality and beauty: one day offering courses on seeking the divine in everyday life, the next trotting out "21 Day Booty Core."

Look at me, I thought. Just a girl in the world, tidying up, doing nothing special, free from the endless self-imposed pressure. I read a little Ralph Waldo Emerson, possibly the world's greatest expert on just living life. "He is rich who owns the day, and no one owns the day who allows it to be invaded by fret and anxiety." Got that right, RWE.

I ate a bag of barbecue potato chips for lunch. I walked the dogs along my usual walk/run route because I didn't feel like running. I deleted some emails because I didn't feel like answering them. I read a novel instead of writing some essay I was supposed to be working on. I ordered a box of overpriced decorative folders that I didn't need from Amazon. I had a glass of wine at 4:30 p.m.

The exhilaration I'd felt earlier in the day began to peter out. I felt a little gassy from my lunch of potato chips. I like to think of myself as a woman with a rich interior life. I read old books and pursue my cockamamie interests. I am a half-assed knitter and an excellent baker of blackberry pies, complete with flawless latticework tops. I ride a motorcycle. I volunteer at a dog rescue and have three dogs of my own. I believed that once I swore off self-improvement it would free up headspace for my other interests. I imagined my interests to be like goldfish, which are said to grow as big as their bowl. Who knows what I might attempt now! But I felt restless and anxious. I bought a subscription to Babbel, the language-learning app. I didn't even open it. Instead, second glass of wine in hand, I found myself scrolling through DailyOM, one of the newsletter subscriptions I had deleted just that morning, to see if there was a gentle, rational regimen that could help me get "back on track."

It turned out swearing off self-improvement was as fraught as launching into a new self-improvement regime. Trying to improve myself had been a form of self-medication, my habitual response whenever something wasn't going the way I wanted it to. I never admitted it, but I felt I would only deserve whatever good thing I was hoping for—true love, a book contract, a body I felt comfortable in—if I was a better woman. I was used to the striving and misery. It was familiar. It was *home*. True Self was a stranger, someone I'd gone to great lengths to pretend didn't exist.

I once married a man in penance for falling in love with someone who was so obviously wrong for me. He was straight-up blue-collar, something I loved about him. He knew how to get up before dawn, work a solid eight hours, arrive home dog-tired and in need of a shower and a beer. It was a confusing time in popular music. Sheryl Crow sang about being a rough-and-ready woman of the people who day drank with strangers in the middle of the week in her halter top and low-rise jeans (in my imagination) and hooked up with truckers in Barstow. All she wanted to do was have some fun. There was another girl singer who sang a more troubling song about getting involved with a sexy cowboy for whom she wears a sexy dress and pours him a cold glass of lemonade; years pass and she's stuck in the kitchen cooking for him and their kids while he goes to the bar (possibly to hook up with Sheryl Crow). That's the one I should have listened to.

My guy wasn't a sexy cowboy but a sexy UPS man. You can laugh. I did, even as it was happening. It made no sense as a love story, but complete sense as a self-improvement story. With this man, who reminded me of all the boys I knew from high school who preferred less difficult girls, I could be the woman my mother thought I should be. The mother I had murdered by not being the kind of daughter she'd hoped for.

For the first time in my life I was thin enough. My doctor did a blood test to see if perhaps I was dying of some hidden disease, but I was only anemic and rocking size 6 jeans. The man had two young children who lived with us. One of their mothers had disappeared, the other lived in another state. I spent days baking elaborate cakes for their birthdays. We went on family outings to county fairs and locally famous waterfalls and caves. I would pack a picnic. He liked me to paint my toenails seafoam green. He liked me to sleep in one of his oversize T-shirts and string bikini underpants, even though I preferred to sleep naked. He liked every crappy science fiction movie that came down the pike, and I endured them because he liked to hold my hand at the movies. At night, after overseeing bath time, story time, and tucking-in time, I read about the Tudors. I went through a mad Elizabeth I phase (another of my cockamamie interests). Meanwhile, he played a video game called EverQuest, which seemed to be set during Elizabeth's reign.

My friends were polite. My best friend said, "But, is this *you*?" By me, she meant True Self, the one I was always trying to abandon in the name of self-improvement, the one my mother believed was too much, and not enough. My best friend knew me to be smart, curious, adventuresome, loathing of domesticity, sardonic. I said, "I don't need to be able to talk about Dostoevsky with him. I have you for that." That hadn't been her question. Later, thinking back, I would note that I leapt straight to what would reveal itself to be the insurmountable problem between us. Several years later, after I had married him and the marriage was in the process of falling apart, I was going to the movies with this same friend. We were going to see *Pollock*. My husband and I had reached that stage where anything was grist for a knock-down, drag-out argument. I baited him. I said, "I'm going with Kathy because I didn't think you'd want to see a movie about Jackson Pollock." He looked blank. I added, ". . . the *artist*." He said, "Oh I see, he's a fucking tortured artist like you?"

The grief at the end of that marriage was grief for love lost. Grief for mother lost. Grief because no matter how hard I tried, I couldn't be the woman my mother felt I needed to be to have what she felt was a good life. Guilt because I wanted to want to be that woman but could not. Guilt because I wanted to want the sort of life I had with this husband, one that I felt my mother would have approved, but I did not. Not really. Not ever.

That calamitous marriage ended in 2000. Now, on the night of the morning I swore off self-improvement in April 2017, I couldn't sleep. This was unusual for me. One of the things I never needed to improve about myself was my capacity for a good night's sleep. During the few weeks I was tethered to my Fitbit, I learned that it took me less than two minutes to fall asleep. Turns out even my half-ass daily exercise routine, consisting of thirty minutes of walking one block then running one block around the neighborhood, helped me sleep well. Clearly, I didn't need to swear *that* off; plus, my walk/run was a break in the day that I truly enjoyed. As I lay in the dark staring up at the ceiling with everyone snoring around me— the three dogs on their respective beds, the husband next to me—I suddenly said, "Huh!" right out loud. I saw how swearing off self-improvement could easily become yet another self-improvement regime. Yeah, no, that was totally not happening. I needed to find another way.

A word about self-improvement versus self-care.

Whether we're hamster-wheeling the self-improvement

program du jour or practicing yeah, no, not happening, we need to take care of ourselves. It's not a special occasion thing we splurge on when we're two steps from a rubber room.

Self-care, in its current benign and twee iteration, is signified in images of overpriced throw pillows marching along the backs of comfy-looking sofas; cups of artisanal hot chocolate served in a mug calligraphed with *Live, Laugh, Love*; and bubble baths with enough pillar candles artfully arranged around the perimeter of the tub to suggest a satanic ritual. So far so good. Not arguing with this message.* It's good to sit on the couch with something warm to drink. It's good to take a bath. We need to do more of it, every day. Full stop.

But most of us don't do this. We find it to be a waste of time. Or we say we'll take a break when everything else is done, but everything is never done—a situation further confused by the value we place on appearing to work ourselves to death. Instead of taking care of ourselves, we whip ourselves into a paroxysm of insomnia and stress-related ailments, self-medicating along the way, until we're on the verge of a breakdown, then collapse into the arms of self-care. This often translates to "treating ourselves" to a girlfriend's getaway, long weekend, or spa package, which brings its own stress—spending money we don't have,

---

* Actually, I am. You know my complicated feelings about expensive candles. In the movies, the broke girl who barely makes ends meet is nevertheless always able to take a bath in her roach-infested apartment surrounded by several hundred dollars' worth of candles.

fretting about how we look in a swimsuit, feeling guilty about taking time off/leaving the spouse and kids to fend for themselves. As often as not, we then come home feeling like we need a vacation from the vacation. The inbox is exploding, the house looks as if it's been ransacked by a covert search team, and the healthy vegetable casserole we guilt-baked before we left hasn't been touched.

In many ways, self-care bills itself as a supplement to self-improvement, but like self-improvement it usually becomes yet another thing we're supposed to be doing and end up failing at.

Writing in the *Los Angeles Times*, Jennifer Conlin reported on her efforts to wedge some self-care into her days. Her life is a not-unfamiliar picture of stress: high-pressure job, husband whose equally stressful job takes him often to perilous parts of the world, one child a senior in college, the others launching new careers in far-flung cities, elderly parents under her own roof and for whom she is the sole caretaker. She needed some "me time," stat! She downloaded a meditation app, signed up for Zumba classes and a once-a-week piano class, and started seeing a therapist.

"Between work, family, travel, and my outside commitments, I started falling further and further behind on my self-imposed schedule," Conlin writes. In her weekly therapy appointment, she discussed her failure to keep up her self-care routine, and her therapist nodded in agreement. "My self-care almost killed me."

We need to take care of ourselves. But here's some good

news! Since we've all been on the receiving end of easily a za-billion "wellness" messages for years, we already have a pretty good idea what it entails. We know how to do this already. If you want to stop feeling like crap when you go to bed, stop eating barbecue potato chips for lunch. If you want to have more stamina, run around the block on a regular basis. When you need to stop, stop. When you need to rest, rest. Get the correct amount of sleep. Drink some water. It's not difficult.

Care for yourself in the way you would a beloved pet. Every day you make sure she gets a nice walk, some good food, and naps. You know her favorite treats and the place behind her ears where she loves to be scratched. You pet her head and talk to her and make her feel loved. Even on a busy day you do this. If you can do this for a pet, you can do this for yourself.

According to Samsung, the average person will take twenty-five thousand selfies in their lifetime. This sounds like a number pulled straight out of the hipster chapeau of some front-facing camera marketing lackey, but no matter. That's a staggering amount of look-at-me-look-at-me right there. We're living in an era of unapologetic self-absorption, which is at the root of our obsession with self-improvement. To short-circuit the self-improvery impulse, we need to cut the connection, focus on something else. And I don't mean your family and their endless needs—chances are one of the things you're also concerned with improving is how to be a better wife and mom, which usually translates to doing more for your family, not less—I mean expanding your knowledge of what it means to be a yeah, no, not happening woman in the world.

One of my first cockamamie—and extremely nerdy—interests was reading *National Geographic* magazine. My parents were longtime subscribers, and their old issues were among my most cherished possessions. About the time I was starting to connect the dots—that the sanctioned lot of females consisted of dusting, vacuuming, grocery shopping, and cooking the nightly meal for people who couldn't care less, and yikes! that would be my lot one day if I wasn't careful—I discovered Amelia Earhart and Jane Goodall. I saw immediately that Amelia and Jane were a different kind of grown-up woman. They didn't seem to spend any time standing in front of the stove, stirring a pot of spaghetti sauce. They didn't drag their plastic laundry baskets to the Laundromat once a week, that I could see. Instead, they threw themselves into the world, and pursued their passions without apology. They devoted their lives to flying airplanes across oceans and studying chimpanzees in Africa. That's what they cared about, and that's what they did. They wanted to be good at doing things that mattered to them.

In college, I went through a mad Gertrude Stein phase. Stein lived in Paris between the wars, collected art, nurtured and sparred with Hemingway, loved Alice B. Toklas, and lived an entire life devoted to not going along with the crowd. Her self-proclaimed masterpiece, the 925-page *The Making of Americans*, remains impenetrable and unreadable, even to the most ardent of Stein scholars. She was hailed as a genius of modernism, even though almost no one could get beyond her most famous observation: "A rose is a rose is a rose is a rose." And that's only because Toklas embroidered it on their tea towels.

I wish I could bottle and sell Stein's moxie, slipping it into the pamplemousse La Croix of every woman I know. Stein had a philosophy class with William James at Radcliffe. He was her favorite professor but when it came time to take the final exam, she wrote him a note on the top of the test paper: "Dear Professor James, I am so sorry but really I do not feel a bit like an examination paper in philosophy today." Then she got up from her desk and went home. The next day she received a postcard from Professor James: "Dear Miss Stein, I understand perfectly how you feel. I often feel like that myself." For having the guts to put her own feelings and desires first, she was awarded the highest grade in the class. Or so the story goes.

Even as a young woman of no importance, Stein was sure about what mattered to her and what didn't. She was born in 1874 and came of age during the era when women of her class were expected to be frail things, spending most of their time in bed with "nervous headaches." Gertrude was stout and hardy and loved hiking in the middle of summer until she had to stop and take a nap on a rock in the shade. She said yeah, no, not happening to heteronormativity, traditional femininity, letting anyone interrupt her while she was working, suffering fools, and punctuation.

This allowed her to say yes to what mattered to her: her work, collecting Picasso (whom nobody was crazy about back then), driving all over the road like a maniac in her Model T Ford, the aforementioned tramping around in the dead of summer, and Alice. She lived a modest life of ease and luxury, all because she said fuck it all to everything that was expected of her and yes to what mattered to her. Stein believed she was a literary genius, but what she is famous for is being a singular woman who built a life that suited her. I wanted to be that kind of woman.

I've become a student of women's soccer star Megan Rapinoe, and the way she lives life on her own terms. Cocaptain of the championship 2019 US women's soccer team, Rapinoe took grief for refusing to censor her opinions or rein herself in for every unapologetic display of triumph. Even though it all seemed girlish, free, and genuinely authentic, when the US team spanked Thailand in the opening round of the 2019 World Cup, she was chided for her behavior.

Aside from her extraordinary athleticism and brilliance on the field, Rapinoe is a hilarious free spirit. After the quarter final match against host country France, which the United States won on her two goals, she freestyled some commentary, "Go gays. You can't win a championship without gays on your team. It's never been done before, ever. That's science, right there." Her incandescent fame predictably has attracted a kaleidoscope of haters. It is to be expected, and she doesn't seem to care. When a woman says fuck it all, there is always pushback. It goes hand in hand with being a competitor; perhaps this is something men have always known. If a woman learns to compete, whether on the sports field or in the market economy, and she learns how to cope with not being liked, look out.

It's instructional that, despite refusing to suppress her personality or apologize for being herself, Rapinoe has managed to sidestep the infamous Likability Trap. In 2019, she won the prestigious Ballon d'Or Féminin, awarded to the most outstanding female soccer star of the year. She was also named *Sports Illustrated*'s Sportsperson of the Year. She graced the December 2019 cover of *SI* in a white Valentino gown (with long sleeves, a turtleneck, a graphic print of pink roses, and an image of a sculpture of a couple locked in a passionate embrace), holding a sledgehammer. Rapinoe's hair is still short and pink, her expression a confident, playful-yet-defiant smirk. If this isn't a cause for optimism, reader, I don't know what is.

Eccentric actress Frances McDormand is also a poster woman for the yeah, no, not happening ethos. McDormand appeared at the 2018 Oscars with finger-combed hair and no makeup, wearing a long-sleeved gold-brown dress that looked as if it were made from the clippings found on the floor of a busy dog groomer. She had just won her second Best Actress Oscar for her performance in *Three Billboards Outside Ebbing, Missouri*. Her appearance signaled that Hollywood's rules were of no interest to her. In her stream-of-consciousness speech she thanked her husband and son, "both feminists," compared her feelings to that of Olympian snowboarder Chloe Kim, who'd just killed it with back-to-back 1080s in the half-pipe, and suggested to the mucky-mucks in the audience that rather than chat insincerely about working together at the after-parties, they finance her projects and those of her fellow nominees. At the end of her forty-five seconds she left the audience with two words: inclusion rider. She dropped a look on the audience that said, "look it up, fools."* Then she picked up her Oscar, which for some reason she had placed on the floor beside her, perhaps so she could gesticulate more freely, curtsied a little sardonically, and left the stage. The *New Yorker* headline reported, "Frances McDormand Makes the Oscars Weird Again."

It may seem silly to collect stories about the lives of famous women as if they were trading cards, but let's not forget the power of mimetic desire, the powerful innate urge to imitate that which we admire.

In those early days of swearing off self-improvement I dumped every habit that didn't serve me, but took care of myself in a habitual, haphazard, nothing-fancy way. An apple a day. A vegetable or two at dinner. A walk/run around the block in the mornings. Resting when I felt like resting. Ignoring my phone at night. I called this good enough. I made no lists, no resolutions, no plans to do anything different.

---

* To save you from googling: an inclusion rider is a clause that any actor can ask to be included in their movie contract, demanding a certain level of diversity in the hiring of cast and crew.

I stopped thinking so much about myself, which was a fucking relief. Instead, I paid attention to women who walked through the world in a way that appealed to me. I reread some of my favorite biographies of remarkable females, paying special attention to how the heroines said yeah, no, not happening. In 2018, I published a book about difficult women. It was an investigation of women from different times and places and the way they disobeyed the rules of their time. In what ways did they refuse to go along to get along? What parts of the stereotype of the ideal female did they disregard? They were a highly flawed, deeply wonderful cadre of sorry-not-sorry, life-is-what-I-make-it human beings.

At first, immersing myself in the lives of women who weren't much interested in self-improvement, who saw nothing wrong with thumbing their noses at a culture unable to prevent their being who they were and doing what they wanted, seemed uninspired. Surveyor Karen and Surveyed Karen tussled with each other. The Surveyor wanted me to leap into action—go to clown school! Become a stunt driver! Throw away all your concealers! The Surveyed pushed back—she wasn't smiling now—wasn't that just another form of self-improvement? Wasn't that just chasing after a new ideal, in this case the new unimproved improved self? Wasn't reading my way through inspiring bios something my True Self enjoyed? The Self who found comfort and support in this not very exciting and frankly nerdy activity? I debated this aloud. I felt as if I were in a one woman play, performed in front of a ten-year-old laptop with cookie crumbs between the keys. I wondered if self-improvement had been a part of my life for so long, I didn't know how to be myself without it.

Permission to follow my instincts arrived in the form of Anne Helen Petersen's *Too Fat, Too Slutty, Too Loud: The Rise and Reign of the Unruly Woman*. Petersen confesses in the introduction that she wanted to write about unruly women to figure out how to become one. "I spent the bulk of my adolescent life internalizing the fact that girls who crossed that invisible line would become pariahs: excised from their communities and families, unable to find work or companionship. I was wrong, of course, but it took finding my own group of weird, confident, *too much* friends for me to lean into my own difference, my own modes of unruliness."

The women I wrote about felt like friends, but I also had one real-life friend who had always been a role model. Kathy, my best friend since graduate school, said fuck it all a long time ago, and doesn't try to fix herself. She is a compulsive reader of nineteenth-century novels, an old-movie fiend, and kind of a slob. She drinks good red wine and smokes (she really should quit, but yeah, no, not happening) and weight-wise is just this side of getting a stern talking-to by her primary care doctor. When she gets drunk, she talks too loud and misremembers the past. She wears nothing but black tank-top dresses that she accessorizes with stacks of cheap bracelets. At any given time, she has just enough money in her checking account to go to France for two weeks. She's had double hip replacements, and on one side there was some nerve damage, and now she wears a brace and a funny shoe. I told her that shit was probably *actionable*. That she could probably sue the doctor who nicked the nerve. She just laughed at me. It would cost far too much time, energy, and money, and anyway the nerve is supposed to grow back before she dies. (Update: it has. Kathy was right.) She has a job as the head of marketing for an arts organization that she loves; her performance review always suggests she up her social media game, to which she says—let's say it together— yeah, no, not happening. She still earns high marks, because everyone loves her and nobody thinks she should be any other way. Kathy is an inspiration. She is light and free. Since she dropped out of the self-improvement rat race, her ability to own her flaws has made her seem both charming and enviable.

When I asked Kathy her secret to self-acceptance she said, "I like myself this way. Plus, being myself is just so much *easier*."

CHAPTER 8

The Yeah, No. Not Happening Cheat Sheet

No matter what you are supposed to do, you can prove the supposition wrong, just by doing something else.

—Mark Greif, *Against Everything*

Saying yeah, no, not happening is about learning to evade the tyranny of culturally sanctioned bullshit. It's about figuring out what you want to do and taking a pass on the rest.

Before we say yes or no to something, we need to take some time to think about it. Our Buy Now with One Click culture discourages taking even a minute for consideration, which is how I wound up with not one but two weighted blankets, an essential oil diffuser, a fruit dehydrator, and a subscription to a webinar that promises to boost creativity while lowering anxiety—I think. I bought it during a low moment when I felt very anxious and uncreative; then the moment passed and I forgot about it.

To be able to say yeah, no, not happening with authority, we've got to seriously entertain what it would mean to say yes. That's why we start with *yeah*, which translates to "okay, I'm going to spend some time thinking about this."

Consider: *where* is this urge to improve yourself coming from? Is the inner Surveyor on your case because you've been too freewheeling lately, reminding you a good modern woman is always disciplined and self-policing? Are you disappointed with the realities of True Self and wanting to escape who you are by resuming the chase after fantasy best self? Did you simply see a product being shilled by a beautiful influencer online and that stirred up all your dissatisfaction, disappointment, and insecurity? Did your mother say something to you on your birthday?

Consider: *why* do you want to say yes? To do something, *anything*, even something lame and expensive, to feel better about yourself and your life? To go along with the other Stepford wives doing radical puppy Pilates?* Because you don't know who you are if you're not improving yourself? Or is it something that True You genuinely requires?

---

* Actually, if that's not a thing it should be.

Consider: *what* does it cost in time and energy? Is there someone who stands to make money from your decision?

If upon reflection you feel like a Wednesday night karaoke date with the women from the office would be a zany break from an otherwise dull workweek, say yeah, it's happening! Likewise, if you have trouble getting enough fruits and veg in your diet and that weekly smoothie delivery service, though a little expensive, would make life easier, go for it. Extreme waxing of your lady bits? Know that I'm saying yeah, no, not happening, and also judging you, but you can tell me to fuck right on off. To each her own, sister.

I hope by now it's clear that the best thing you can do to improve your life is to say a hard no to most of the self-improvement-related nonsense being thrust upon us every minute of every day. Anything that will eventually make you feel like crap about yourself: no. Anything that feeds self-doubt while eroding your ability to trust your knowledge and instincts: no. Anything that features a moving goalpost: no and no. Saying no signals that we respect our own judgment, our time and energy. We're setting boundaries when we say no. We're practicing self-respect.

Saying not happening underscores this. It turbo powers your no. It seals the deal. No, this is totally not happening. Added bonus, it makes you sound confident in your decision, especially to your own ears.

Gentle reader, below is a list of some of the most common situations to which we would all do well to say yeah, no, not happening. This list is not comprehensive but represents popular arenas of self-improvery that I wish would disappear immediately, along with rompers for men.

If you're so inclined, I would be thrilled if you would join me in saying yeah, no, not happening to:

Anti-Aging Anxiety

Remember Kim Novak's 2014 Oscar appearance? Best known for her role in Alfred Hitchcock's *Vertigo*, she was considered one of the great beauties of her time. For the last few decades she's lived on a ranch near Rogue River, Oregon, which is to say in seclusion. She was delighted to have been asked to present and did what every woman in the known world would have done—tried to look her best. For which she was burned at the Twitter stake. Mostly men piled on, making jokes about sending her back to the wax museum. But there were plenty of hateful women: Why does Kim Novak look like she had a face transplant? She reminds me of a jack-o'-lantern. Why? *Why?* Because the woman was eighty-one years old and was doing what all women over forty do these days: everything we can to look a young, dewy twenty-five.

The turnstile of life goes but one way. You are older now than you were when you read the last sentence. It's the reality of human existence, a biological certainty. And yet, aging women are despised, both for looking older and for trying to do what they can to not look old. The only escape from this is to say fuck it all. The only way to take back your power is to say yeah, no, not happening.

As with all things, there is balance. No one is saying you're required to look like the Crypt Keeper in the name of living as your most authentic self. (My most authentic self looks like a hearty, aging Eastern European peasant woman with better-than-average bone structure.)

Say yeah, no, not happening to what doesn't work for you. Resolve to do what you do. Don't make a religion out of it. Want to dye your hair? Great. Do more push-ups than a marine? Fine, whatever. Tend to your beauty in whatever way feels right to you and say yeah, no, not happening to everything else.

Anything that Includes Getting Up at Some Godforsaken Hour

I think I've failed to stand up enough for New Age woo. I'm a fellow traveler. I've done my share of meditation. I've gone to a yoga retreat in a foreign land. I've seen my share of psychics, shamans, and astrologers. I'm intrigued and feel as if life is made richer by it (because I'm a Pisces, all right?), but I am in no way getting up in the dark to practice any of this shit. In our rush to pack more into every day, not only have we lost respect for our need to sleep, but we've also somehow decided to disregard the science of circadian rhythms, which determines our chronotype, or personal body clock. Some people are hardwired to get up early; some are hardwired to stay up late. And yet, we're living in weirdly puritanical times, when to get up early for a 6:00 a.m. yoga class signals the correct amount of devotion to spiritual questing, self-care, and firm triceps.

The time you awaken in the morning is not a referendum on your depth or devotion to soul and self. Say yeah, no, not happening to feeling guilty for owning your night-owl nature.

Believing Happiness Is Out of Reach Because You Don't Have a Nice Ass

The irony of living a life devoted to self-improvement is that we believe we're doing it to be happy, which only serves to confirm our fundamental assumption that we don't deserve to be happy right this minute. The lie we're told by consumer culture is that only the Ideal Female deserves happiness. You know the rest: since it's impossible to attain this ideal, it's impossible to be truly happy.

In 2006, Duke University conducted a study on happiness. Eight universal traits of happy people were identified. Notice, please, that none of them have anything to do with wellness, detoxing, exfoliating, working out, cardio, decluttering, organizing the hall closet, or even finding true love.

1. Lack of suspicion and resentment
2. Not living in the past
3. Not wasting time and energy fighting things you cannot change
4. Staying involved with the world
5. Refusing to indulge in self-pity
6. Cultivating old-fashioned virtues (love, compassion, humor, loyalty)
7. Not expecting too much of yourself
8. Finding something bigger than yourself to believe in (self-centered people scored lowest in any test measuring happiness)

To spend our days consumed by tracking and measuring, in the hopes that we will one day be thin enough, fit enough, mindful enough, productive enough, charitable enough, kind enough to earn the right to be happy is utter crap. Say yeah, no, not happening to all that, and yes to the Buddhist wisdom that solves the happiness problem in four words: Want what you have.

Caring Too Much about Being Liked

As the tenders and befrienders of the species, women are more susceptible to feeling unhappy when they feel disliked. As we've established, being disliked makes us feel judged, which triggers shame, which launches us into our next self-improvery program, the one that is going to make us everyone's favorite. It should be noted that this isn't a universal response. My Polish grandmother, my father's mother, fully expected not to be liked by everyone. She wanted to be loved by the few people she loved. Otherwise, she felt that being disliked was a mark of character; to be liked by everyone signaled you were a people pleaser, which made you both uninteresting and, paradoxically, unlikable.

As we saw in chapter 3, the most easily likable women are those who are devoted to improving themselves, which signals an agreeable lack of confidence in who they are. They work on looking prettier and younger, and also strive to improve their organizational skills and productivity, so that they can do more for others. The moment they accept themselves for who they are—how uppity, how arrogant—or are suspected of improving themselves in the name of ambition or self-interest, they become unlikable. Likewise, if they're too opinionated, by which I mean having opinions.

Jessica Valenti sums up the reality of living to be liked in the *Nation*: "Wanting to be liked means being a supporting character in your own life, using the cues of the actors around you to determine your next line rather than your own script. It means that your self-worth will always be tied to what someone else thinks about you, forever out of your control."

We regain control the moment we swear off prioritizing the

approval of others over inhabiting our True Selves. The more we step into who we are, the more we swear off self-improvement, the greater chance we have of gaining the confidence to say take me as I am, a genuine expression of self-love.

Complicating the Simple Act of Drinking Water for Fuck's Sake

Say yeah, no, not happening to Waterlogged, Hydro Coach, iHydrate, and all the rest of those hydration apps. And while we're at it, all the other digital hand-holders that train you not to trust your own body. We imagine we're taking better care of ourselves by constantly monitoring basic human functions, but we're contributing to our own enfeeblement. We're voluntarily alienating ourselves from our selves. The message we're sending ourselves, hour by hour, is that we have no confidence in how our body feels. We develop the habit of feeling disappointed in the limitations of our humanity.

It should be obvious, but apparently it's not: our human bodies are wondrous, complex, and reliable. Why on earth do we think some nerd living on Hot Pockets and Red Bull, noodling away in some split-level start-up accelerator in a Silicon Valley suburb, hoping to strike it rich with his dumb app, knows more about what's good for your body *than your own body*? If you struggle with self-doubt—and who doesn't?—outsourcing simple behaviors and goals to random health-monitoring apps only reinforces it. Free your thirst. Uninstall the apps and every time you pass a sink, have a glass of water.

Denying Our Feelings, Even the So-Called Toxic Ones

Our shadow sides aren't quite so shadowy when we're not trying so bloody hard to be forever full of light, love, joy, extreme kindness, radical empathy, and all the other good and pure traits that seem to follow the Ideal Female throughout the ages. We are still, in many ways, the Angel in the House. Not submissive to men, perhaps, but certainly submissive to the cultural imperative to be charming, graceful, kind, tolerant, and self-sacrificing.

If I could instantly disappear one word from the English language, it would be *toxic*, except as it pertains to bathroom cleanser and pollutants in the environment. Truly hilarious self-help websites offer advice on banishing all toxic emotions. Once you stop allowing fear, envy, shame, frustration, guilt, jealousy, and anger into your life, you will be happy!

You know what's toxic? Being led to believe you can't handle feeling these very human feelings that we all feel. Do you know who successfully avoids feeling these so-called toxic feelings? People who are medicated out of their gourds. They don't feel *anything.*

A good training ground for surviving unpleasant feelings is a cross-country flight during thunderstorm season. Part of the flight will be smooth, and you'll look out the window at the sun reflected off a tower of white clouds and tear up a little because the world is so beautiful. Ten minutes later you'll be jouncing around in your seat and the overhead bins will start popping open and you'll pee your pants a little in terror. I hate to fly, and this is the moment I always ask if I can hold the hand of the person sitting next to me. I've held hands with grandfathers, bloggers, paramedics, software engineers, an orthopedic nurse, an Olympic sprinter, and, on a flight to LA, a rapper.

When I told them I was afraid, and asked if I could hold their hand, all of them said yes. All of them.

This is why we can swear off denying the full spectrum of our feelings with confidence. Because if you ask, there will be someone to help you.

Depriving Yourself of Joy Because of What You Imagine You Look Like

There's a corner of the deep south of France where everybody really is a beach body. The wide and wobbly fleshed show up in their Speedos and string bikinis and no one bats an eye. Women of every shape and size, with every shape and size of breast, fling off their tops, whistle while they slather themselves with suntan oil, and talk loudly on their phones. They seriously have said *tout foutre*. One midweek day in late fall I swam there with some American friends. There was no one else on the beach but us. The sea was clear and warm, the sun high in the sky. Everyone dove in, except for the most beautiful, slender one among us. She sat on the beach with a towel wrapped around her waist, watching. Later, she confessed that she had slept too late that morning, skipped her five-mile run, and indulged in a croissant with raspberry jam for breakfast. Thus, she couldn't possibly expose her body, even (especially) in front of her friends.

She regrets this about herself. She's trying to find a way to feel freer in her body. Sometimes she's able to overcome her self-consciousness, and sometimes her self-consciousness triumphs. Know this too: part of saying yeah, no, not happening is also accepting that you can't say it all the time.

The degree to which no one is looking at us is really quite stunning. We're all too busy staging and snapping our selfies. Most of the time when we fret about our muffin tops, chin zit, or hair frizz, no one is paying attention. Once, I put on a pair of jeans that had a pair of underpants stuck in one leg. When I was on stage, ready to give a talk, they fell out. I quickly swooped down, picked them up, and stuffed them in my back pocket. Everyone was so busy looking at their screens they didn't even notice.

Our feelings about our bodies are so personal, and we are so judgmental, of ourselves and others. But it's always worth the struggle to choose joy rather than giving in to fear about how we appear. I firmly believe this urge to cut loose is ingrained;

THE YEAH, NO. NOT HAPPENING CHEAT SHEET

look no further than the colossal success of the terrible movie *Mamma Mia!*

Detoxing, as We're Calling Dieting Now, Apparently

Any eating plan that requires a degree in biochemistry to make lunch? Yeah, no, not happening. A full examination of our demented and complicated relationship with food is above my pay grade, but I invite you to swear off any complicated eating plan that tries to brainwash you into thinking a square of mashed cashews is an acceptable substitute for cheese. None of the celebrity-sanctioned diets—paleo, the Zone, raw food, Atkins, keto—fared well in the 2019 *U.S. News & World Report* rankings. And I beg of you, just because *U.S. News* is depressingly fogey-ish, and not sexy in the manner of your favorite IG microinfluencer pictured biting into a homemade paleo chocolate chip cookie, clad only in an oversize sweatshirt fetchingly falling off one slender shoulder, that has no bearing on the facts.

In *Secrets from the Eating Lab: The Science of Weight Loss, the Myth of Willpower, and Why You Should Never Diet Again,* psychologist Traci Mann reminds us that diets don't work for the obvious reason that eating is a matter of self-preservation. Three completely rotten biological changes occur when we restrict food. The first is neurological: food starts to look more delicious and irresistible. The second change is hormonal: as you lose weight, the hormones that contribute to a feeling of fullness decrease, while those that signal hunger increase. The third change is metabolic: your metabolism becomes more efficient, which makes it even harder to lose weight.

If you want to find and maintain your best weight, follow the famous Michael Pollan directive: Eat food, not too much, mostly plants.

But that's not what bedevils us, is it? The larger problem is that for women in the modern world, losing weight always pairs nicely with every other self-improvement regime. It has *always* accompanied every other self-improvement program I've undertaken. Being thinner fixes everything. Whatever else needs to be fixed, losing weight—now reframed as "detoxing" or clean eating—can always be added to the self-improvery menu. Get more organized and lose weight. Spend more quality time with family and lose weight. Be more mindful and lose weight.

Extreme Workouts That Lead to Vomiting

Making a religion out of working out makes me cranky. When how hard and long we "train" becomes yet another avenue for virtue-signaling, I become even more unbearable. How is it that unless we're maintaining a workout regime on par with an Olympic gymnast, world-class tennis player, or Madonna, we're made to feel like hopeless couch potatoes, even if we are getting in movement every day?

I'm not going to bag on CrossFit (okay, I am a little), but the insider lingo, cultish "community," and shaming of everyone who doesn't see the magic of working out until you want to die is *no bueno*.

Instead, I prefer to take the advice of my glamorous aunt Jackie, for whom fitness was sidestroking three lengths of the swimming pool, then settling down in a chaise longue with a highball and a cigarette in a gold cigarette holder: "Go run around the block." Advice I still take. Be right back.

Choose an activity that causes you to break a sweat, and do it a few times a week. It doesn't matter what it is, and it's not necessary to take it up a notch. Indeed, there are no longer any notches, just showing up and moving around. I like someone to boss me around in the realm of fitness. Even the worst exercise class is good if it features someone standing at the front of the room barking orders. I've tried exercising in front of a mirror, where I order myself to do fifteen squats, and it just doesn't work. My standards are very low, exercise-wise, and I've learned to say yeah, no, not happening to raising them. As long as I do enough to keep my blood pressure within a healthy range and avoid extreme kimono arms, I'm good.

Of course, if you're an avid sportswoman, you should say yeah, no, not happening to *my* pathetic bullshit and go about your business.

Fanatical Goal-Setting

Goals, like hydration, are a fetish for our times. Ten years down the road, it will undoubtedly be something else. Fanatical goal-setting is usually indistinguishable from fanatical self-improvery, number one on the list of yeah, no, not happening. Setting fanatical goals related to our bodies—weight, dress size, a specific cut of jean we'd like to rock at the high school or family reunion—are a surefire way to set ourselves up for failure and activate the self-improvement spiral of guilt/shame/new program to "get on track."

I very unscientifically polled half a dozen friends over margaritas about what they're trying to improve, and it appears goal-setting is the new diet culture. In the same way planning to go on a diet on Monday is the best way to ensure you'll eat an entire cheesecake on Sunday night, extreme goal-setting has a way of creating the perfect climate for rebelling against the very goal that you've set. Read more literature turns into watch more TV. Get up earlier becomes sleeping even later because you're so pissed at yourself and depressed for not getting up at the mandated time.

Possibly my friends are as goal-resistant as I am, but hauling out your million-dollar planner (see productivity) and writing down thirty-seven achievable goals, breaking them into smaller, achievable, measurable segments, breaking those into—God, it's so boring just typing this I can't even continue. Unless spreadsheets and micromanaging your every move make your panties damp, please say yeah, no, not happening to all this hyper self-vigilance. If you must always be working toward a goal, make it one that speaks to your heart and you can keep in your head, then do it.

Idolizing Badassery

Being a badass is one of the twenty-first century's most popular trends in self-remodeling.* The badass bitch is the twin sister of the cool girl: confident and passionate, they're fearless extroverts who set boundaries like a boss and never shrink from a challenge. They've never met a zip line, rock-climbing wall, or tequila shot they didn't like. They're badass! They're also simply the newest iteration of the Ideal Female. The badass bitch is to the twenty-first century what the frail, sickly Angel in the House was to the late nineteenth.

I wouldn't be surprised if the badass bitch is so not you. For one thing, you're reading a book, not diving with sharks off Costa Rica. What if you're a shy introverted chick who is at her best obeying the Girl Scout law? What if you're an observer of life and not an attention-grabber in a leather jacket? What if you think small-batch mezcal is overrated and you're happy with a nice glass of chardonnay, even though your friends tease

---

* You can also have a big ass, as large booties are also in vogue. Thanks to the Kardashians, silicone butt implants are the fastest-growing plastic surgery procedure in the United States.

you for being boring? Aspiring to be a badass is just a different form of suffocating social expectation that can lead you down the well-worn path of "never good enough."

When all that tough chick advice comes rolling at you like a *Raiders of the Lost Ark* boulder? Say yeah, no, not happening. Staying with what you know to be true about yourself, even if it's not in vogue, is the *real* badass move.

Overparenting

This one's tricky, because most of us will do *anything* for our kids. It's all "Yes, of course, everything is happening for you, Little Tomato!" We parents share a variation on the motto of the Los Angeles Police Department: to protect and to serve and to make sure you never suffer the wrath of your algebra teacher because you didn't do your homework.

On the list of female societal pressures: Be a Great Mom is number two, after Be Thin and Sexy at All Times. It's a completely impossible metric.

From *Parents* magazine: "Stressed? 28 Ways to Unwind—By Tonight!" (Yes, there's a fucking deadline.) Also, it's suggested you do this not because you're a raving lunatic from the stress of being all things to all people all the time, but "for the whole family." Meaning: unwinding is yet another thing you're doing for someone else. I can't even with this.

"Laugh" is the first command. And if you don't feel in the

mood to laugh, you're supposed to ask yourself, "If a friend were telling me this story, would I laugh?" (Presumably this is related to a toddler smearing poop on the living room wall.)

My friend Diana is the poster mom for sane parenting. She's raised three boys who are well-rounded, kind, and independent, while also writing, traveling, investing in real estate, and buying and refurbishing a historic bar on the Oregon coast. Plus, she seems to enjoy life. She never looks as if she's one birthday party away from a nervous breakdown.

First, she said yeah, no, not happening to all the stuff that comes with parenting. Before she was pregnant she traveled in India, where she watched mothers sling their babies in trees using a sari while they worked in the fields. That was a clear indication to her that you didn't need to buy out Babies R Us to actually raise a baby. You could get by with diapers and a set of working boobs.

She relied on her own judgment and simple maternal logic. "When I wanted to hold my babies when they cried, I did. I thought my friends who were reading books about getting babies to sleep through the night or on a schedule was bullshit. It would make them ache to hear their babies cry themselves into a fit and I was like, 'It'll pass. They won't cry forever. Hold them!' I felt that my feelings as a parent were natural, so I let them out. I sometimes screamed, I sometimes put myself in time-outs, I cried right in front of them. It seemed like being human is what they were supposed to learn. So, I acted like a complicated female human. Because I am."

As her sons have grown, she's made sure they have some solid life skills, but has otherwise stayed out of their way. She wants them to make their own mistakes, while they're still around for her and their dad to offer help. She wants them to be able to be responsible for their own paperwork, to know how to fill out an employment application and go on a job interview, and to go on a date. When her eldest turned eighteen, he biked from Rome to London. The family called it his launching into adulthood trip. "He texted me from the shores of Dunkirk while looking at England across the Channel. We talked about soldiers his age standing at the ready to fight in World War II and here he was on his bike, as free as he could be." It's a good thing to step back and let our kids make their own way.

Choose your parenting model—reduce it by half, and to the rest say yeah, no, not happening. The unsung benefit to this is that you will be modeling confidence to your children. You don't want them to grow up to be slaves of the culture and, if they're girls, at the beck and call of everyone, do you?

Wallowing in Regret

Once I'd finally more or less sworn off self-improvement, I had a moment (more like a month) of wallowing in regret. Saying fuck it all to the pressure to improve myself freed me *now*, but what about all the years I'd lost by caring way too much? All the diets launched and blown, all the self-second-guessing, all

178

the dumbing down of myself so as not to scare inferior men away, all the dull, misguided dates (and one catastrophic marriage), all the anguish and packages of Nutter Butters when I learned that people I didn't even like didn't like me.

I had a little party before I moved to France and asked everyone what they regretted most in their lives.

Getting married straight out of college, rather than traveling; staying in Germany after college instead of coming home to the love of my life. Staying with my ex-husband because I was afraid no one else would love me; leaving someone I loved because I was afraid he would hurt me. Getting married; not getting married. Becoming a nurse, a lawyer; not going to medical school, not going to law school. Not being able to love myself more. Not seeing how beautiful I was when I was young. Caring too much what people thought of me. Pretending to care about things I didn't really care about. Trying too hard to please everyone around me.

Interestingly, no one regretted a single tattoo.

One woman said, "I have no regrets, only material."

I regret not having thought of that one.

We could make ourselves completely crazy revisiting our past, and sometimes we do just that. It's unrealistic to imagine that we won't fall into a funk one late autumn evening, drink too much, and cry a little about what we imagine might have been. Something to remember, however: if you had made different choices, there's no guarantee you would have been any happier. Because you don't know how marrying the guy or not marrying him, or staying or going, or doing or not doing would have turned out. Conversely, every good thing about your life right now came about because you made the choices you say you regret.

In the end, it's best to give yourself a deadline for wallowing. Listen to some Adele, have a good cry, pass out with your clothes on, and start fresh in the morning. Say yeah, no, not happening to beating yourself up for being human.

Worshipping at the Altar of Productivity

I have no doubt that you're productive enough. Possibly you have two jobs, two children, and a husband whose idea of productivity is folding a basket of clean socks while watching the playoffs. And good on him! That's exactly the level of productivity you should aspire to. The push to do as much as possible in a single day is behind your headaches and insomnia, not the fact that you ate a taco and skipped spin class. You probably needed that taco and a nap. Your body was crying out: "Woman, put down that fucking list, eat some fat and protein, and get some rest!"

You say you feel guilty if you're not maximizing every waking moment? Be aware that that's exactly where mass culture wants you: working your ass off, then buying stuff you don't need to self-soothe.

The best thing you can do for yourself and your family is

help the rest of the crew be at least half as productive as you are. News flash: kids can and should do chores. Their ancestors used to work twelve hours a day on the farm or in the factory; they can fucking load the dishwasher.

Make a to-do list on a piece of paper, then do it. (Yeah.) The hundred-dollar planner with daily affirmations and special boxes and a satin reader's ribbon? (No.) The five-day seminar that features heretofore unknown "hacks"? A waste of time—the exact thing you're trying to combat—and thus, not happening.

I realize this cheat sheet might be a bit daunting. It's not easy to accept our limitations. It's not easy to accept ourselves. It's not easy to suffer an accidental glimpse of ourselves in the selfie camera without wanting to run straight into the arms of the nearest plastic surgeon. It's hard to give up on the completely unrealistic dream of swimming to Cuba, or, you know, running a 5K with your dog on St. Patrick's Day. And it takes courage to let your kid fail because she couldn't look up from her phone long enough to realize everyone else was taking a math test that day.

Bear in mind that small changes, over time, can yield big results.

Practice saying yeah, no, not happening to things that don't matter much and that you really don't want to do. If you honestly can't think of anything you don't want to do, because it's easier just to say yes and make everyone happy and get it over with, start very small. If it still makes your heart race, start even smaller.

If something is just not your thing and you know it's not your thing (costume parties, bed-and-breakfasts, block parties, embroidered pillows with inspirational sayings, goat yoga, any yoga, yogurt), say thanks for thinking of me and decline.

If you don't know whether it's your thing, but you can't see any return in it, other than avoiding the risk of disappointing someone by saying no (taking on all the birthday-party planning at work because having a vagina makes you uniquely qualified, cohosting the neighborhood garage sale, chairing the school auction, naked zip-lining). Um, let me see. Yeah, no. Not happening.

It's ninety-seven degrees at 6:00 p.m. and your nearest and dearest wants to go to the cheap sushi place for dinner? Yeeahhhhhhh, no. Not happening.

"Honey, a guy at work gave me free passes to the twenty-four-hour Best Worst Movie Marathon." Yeah, no. Totally not happening.

Look, black vegan "nice" cream with activated charcoal! Yeah, no.

It's twofer Saturday at the tattoo school. Yeah, uh.

It doesn't have to be anything meaningful to you. In fact, it should be meaningless. The point is to say yeah, no, not happening in a way that feels right, so you can develop your yeah, no, not happening muscle. You can see for yourself that saying yeah, no, not happening isn't going to cause you to lose friends or estrange family members. There's a lot of room for self-expression in the phrase. You can take a page from French and start off with *uhhhhh*, to sort of break the news that you're about to say no. It's a long enough phrase to allow you to put your hand on the question asker's arm. You can even smile when you say it. You will experience firsthand how saying no with love and boundaries is not so difficult after all.

CHAPTER 9

Why Yes, and . . .

The formula of happiness and success is just being actually yourself, in the most vivid possible way you can.

—Meryl Streep

What happens after you stop devoting so much time to self-
improvement, after you say fuck it all and eat a giant carni-
tas burrito with extra sour cream, stay up late reading a thick
biography of Frida Kahlo, skip obligatory and torturous "gatherings," stop forcing yourself to watch the prestige show du
jour because it's a load of pretentious twaddle, stop pretending
to care about your sister's kitchen remodel, stop texting your
college sophomore to make sure he turned in his paper on the
Teapot Dome Scandal, while spending more time hanging out
with friends, napping, catching up on thrillers, walking the
dog around the neighborhood, building a prized collection of
succulents, or otherwise indulging in some eccentric passion
that serves no purpose other than giving you pleasure? What

happens after you've coaxed True Self out of hiding and send phony-baloney best self packing?

You've gotten your social media under control by blocking the sponsored ads and unfollowing the FLEBs and micro-influencers whose lives make you feel like crap. You've freed yourself from best-self dysmorphia disorder by becoming acquainted and making peace with True Self. You've realized that all women receive the message that they are too much and not enough, which only serves to keep us feeling bad about ourselves and endlessly self-improving, buying stuff we don't need that only makes other people rich. You've minimized the time, energy, and money you spend on the fourth shift. You've figured out how to take care of True Self in a way that you can maintain, and you've started hanging out with other women who are living their best fuck-it-all lives. You've sworn off self-improvement, have learned to say fuck it all with verve and sass, and are a model citizen of Yeahnonothappeningville.

Now what?

Stanford professor emerita Patricia Ryan Madson tells a story about her first teaching job. With a graduate degree in theater, she was hired as an assistant professor at Denison University in Ohio. Madson was a smart girl and a good girl. By her own admission, she was a firm believer in "going by the script," and to earn tenure, her most cherished dream, she followed the script to the letter. For a woman in academia, this meant being accommodating, cheerful, and doing more than her share. While teaching nine classes, she volunteered, served on committees, and took a "prestigious assignment" as director of a regional university arts organization. She befriended the right people, filled the gaps and patched the holes, and was the best utility player in the department. She even won an award for her teaching. And yet, when the time came, she was denied tenure. Reason given: that her teaching "lacked intellectual distinction."

After Madson recovered from the heartbreak, she realized that she was surprised but not shocked. She knew she had never taken a chance in her work, never heeded an impulse that might have led to an exciting discovery. She thought this was the end of her academic career, but instead Penn State offered her an assistant professorship in their drama department, teaching voice and acting. Grateful for a do-over, Madson promised herself that this time she would only make choices that felt true to herself. She would only try to make friends with people she liked, would only sit on committees that interested her. She would spend her free time—she had free time now that she wasn't so focused on getting ahead and volunteering for everything—traveling and studying tai chi and pursuing whatever new passions she stumbled upon. Two years later Stanford University offered her a position as director of their undergraduate acting program.

Madson recounts all this in her slim 2005 guide to living, *Improv Wisdom: Don't Prepare, Just Show Up*. By the time she took up the reins at Stanford, she was deep into the world of improv. When most of us think of improv we think of Robin Williams going off on one of his genius rants, or *Whose Line Is It Anyway?*

where the troupe, led by Wayne Brady, is passing around a toilet brush and trying to come up with (hilarious) alternative uses.

Improv as applied to life by Madson is the love child of the Upright Citizens Brigade Theatre and Eastern philosophy. It's about jettisoning overplanning, entering each moment just as you are, finding freedom in the no-pressure attitude of being average and feeling free to make mistakes. It's not surprising, given the outcome of her experience at Denison, where she did everything that was expected of her and was still refused, that she embraced the power of just showing up.

I emailed Madson to tell her that I am one of her biggest fans, to enumerate in embarrassing detail how often I've given *Improv Wisdom* away as a gift, which necessitated purchasing another copy for myself, and also to ask her how we might adapt improv wisdom for the compulsive urge to improve ourselves.

She wrote: "Eventually it becomes clear that any mania for self-improvement is unwarranted and a waste of time. We are so hopelessly self-absorbed. That's the deep problem. One of the reasons that improv is a helpful fix is that it trains the mind to focus outward on what *others* are doing and saying and indicating. You simply cannot improvise if you are thinking up interesting things to do or say. I start my classes by loudly announcing: the important thing you need to know about improv is 'it is not about *you*.'"

It's tricky to say yes, and . . . in a world ruled by the internet.
 Yes and . . .

. . . let me watch just one more dog video, rewatch the installments of James Corden's carpool karaoke (Michelle Obama!), quickly retake all the quizzes that reveal which *Game of Thrones* character I am (I keep getting Daenerys Targaryen, yikes), and catch up on my friend's cooking-school adventures in Tuscany.

Jenny Odell, digital artist and author of *How to Do Nothing: Resisting the Attention Economy*, makes a convincing case for regrounding ourselves in the physical world, for taking the time to "do nothing" as a way of resisting the forces that gobble up our time and attention. The same case can be made for doing nothing as an antidote to the urge to self-improve.

Based in Oakland, every day Odell goes to a local public rose garden, where she sits on a bench and watches birds. She has become a mad bird-watcher, something she never expected. In a lecture she gave concerning her work, she said, "Observing birds requires you quite literally to do nothing. It's sort of the opposite of looking something up online. You can't really look *for* birds. You can't make a bird come out and identify itself to you. All you can do is walk and wait until you hear something, and then stand motionless under a tree trying to use your animal senses to figure out where and what it is. In my experience, time kind of stops. (You can ask anyone who knows me—doing this regularly makes me late to things.)"

There is no reason for Odell to do this, other than it feels good to pay attention.

Saying yes, and . . . makes life the grand adventure it should be, where we're surprised and enriched by the variety of what's out there in the physical world. It's everything happening around us that we've been too self-absorbed to notice. Simple things that make us feel good about being alive. The things to which people who've received a terminal diagnosis start paying attention. News flash: you don't have to wait!

When we're in thrall to self-improvement we do so much that doesn't feel good. We have the aerobics movement of the 1980s to thank for Jane Fonda's mantra "feel the burn," where unless you're holding back tears while exercising it's considered a waste of time. Likewise, the masochistic nature of all pure and holy eating regimens. If, when downing that bright green smoothie, you fail to experience a slight gag reflex, you're not eating clean enough. Kombucha. High colonics. Those knobby foam rollers for "deep tissue massage" that have been outlawed by the Geneva Convention. Yeah, no, so totally not happening.

Factor in our screen addictions, where we live hunched over in the 2-D world, squinting at our phones for hours on end, and the simple human joy of living in our five senses, available to all of us at every minute of the day, is diminished if not forgotten. Diane Ackerman, writing in *A Natural History of the Senses*, calls our world sense-luscious. "When I go biking, I repeat a mantra of the day's sensations: bright sun, blue sky, warm breeze, blue jay's call, ice melting, and so on. This helps me transcend the traffic, ignore the clamorings of work, leave all the mind theaters behind, and focus on nature instead. I still must abide by the rules of the road, of biking, of gravity. But I am mentally far away from civilization. The world is breaking someone else's heart."

You can self-administer a squirt of joy by tuning in to what you're hearing, smelling, feeling, tasting, and seeing right this minute. I'm working in a tiny apartment in the south of France. Outside, past our terrace, with its white enamel tables and tiny metal chairs, I see terra-cotta roofs of different heights and angles, reminding me that Picasso began his cubist phase in this part of the world. A pair of mourning doves are sitting on a chimney. The sky is blue, with a few high white clouds like delicate scarves. I hear the burble of French at the Wednesday farmers market and the laughter of the young woman who works at the nougat shop on the ground floor of our building. She laughs all day long, and when she laughs, I find myself smiling. I can smell the butter in the croissants baking at the boulangerie across the street. The chair I'm sitting on is one of those tiny metal chairs from the terrace. My large American ass is not built for such a chair and my back is killing me. Tuned in to our senses, the imperfection of life around us reminds us of our role in it. It reminds us there is no need to improve anything. (Except possibly my desk chair.)

The irony of the eternal quest for self-improvement is that not only is the experience tedious, but it also shuts down our imagination. There's a lot of talk about imagining a better you, but unless that better you fits into the current culturally approved stereotype of womanhood, you are at risk of believing you've improved nothing. If we don't say yes, and . . . to opportunities that come along that don't fit in with our images of our perfect selves, we pass up the chance to find out something new about ourselves, something we never expected. We miss out on the adventure of self-discovery.

Not long after I swore off self-improvement, I received an email from the Great Pyrenees Rescue Society (GPRS). We had adopted two giant shedding machines from them a few years earlier, Penny and Desmond.* They were Great Pyrenees/Labrador retriever mutts, rescued from a kill shelter in Texas, where Desmond was born. Penny's saga was like the hokiest country and western song: she was a stray who was picked up by the dog catcher after she'd broken her leg. In the kill shelter (dogs have one week before they're euthanized), she had a small litter of puppies. The GPRS pulled Penny and her puppies from the shelter, and all of them died of parvo but Desmond.

The GPRS is based in a suburb of Houston. It's run by a hardworking, no-nonsense doctor's daughter and staffed completely by volunteers. Great Pyrenees are known escape artists, can climb over a five-foot fence, and can dig a hole in your backyard big enough to bury a basketball player in under a minute. The dogs are always getting out and running away. Or

---

* When I took them on walks people asked whether we named them after the devoted lovers Penny Widmore and Desmond Hume in *Lost*. We most certainly did not. On the show Penny and Desmond are long-lost lovers; our Penny is Desmond's mother. They were named after the Beatles songs "Penny Lane" and "Ob-La-Di, Ob-La-Da," featuring Desmond Jones.

people leave them by the side of the road. Or people move and leave the dog tied up to a tree. It's always raining Pyrs in Texas. Twice a month, a transport van departs Texas for the Pacific Northwest, where dogs ready to be adopted are fostered before being placed with their forever families. The email I received from GPRS that day was asking for volunteers to foster. Before I swore off self-improvement this is not something I would have done. I was too busy. I had daily workouts, an ongoing battle with the kitchen and trying to find a way to care about cooking when I did not, my bullet journal and my regular journal, my failing meditation practice. Writing teacher Natalie Goldberg said writing in your journal could also be considered meditation, but that felt like cheating.

I'm embarrassed to admit this, but my fantasy best self also was too urbane and intellectual to be part of a dog rescue, much less one based in *Texas*. Best self was a slender literary writer sitting in a Parisian café in dark-wash jeans and tall boots, somehow also smoking, which I didn't do. She was never hungry and had a flat stomach; she was serene, accomplished, an effortless cook, and a fluent speaker of French.* Her smooth curls escaped from beneath a—I don't know, some kind of an attractive hat. The best-self fantasy insisted on a hat, even though I would have to have a head transplant to wear one without looking like a Polish bowling champion in mourning.

---

* Oh my God, who the fuck is this boring woman?

Now that I had sworn off self-improvement and dumped this best self, I was all in. Without a moment's thought I wrote back and said yes, and . . . what else can I do to help?

We fostered a dog, whom we ended up adopting as well (the aforementioned Rita, with whom I play Dead Hand first thing in the morning). I went on to become a screener, helping to evaluate applications and place the right dog in the right household. People routinely assume Great Pyrenees are white golden retrievers. Nothing could be further from the truth. Pyrs are an ancient livestock guardian dog, bred to live outside with their flocks all year long. Their independent nature makes them difficult to train—they really don't care about your crappy-ass Costco treat—however, they will stand up on their hind legs and eat an entire pot roast off the counter. If you leave your back gate unlatched for two seconds, a dozing Pyr will crack an eye, see his means of escape, nose it open with his strong muzzle, and gallop into the sunset.

The GPRS volunteers are stay-at-home moms, Realtors, nurses, dog trainers, and veterans. They're Christians and atheists, Democrats and Republicans, well-educated and not so much. The great divide that is depressing everyone in the nation does not seem to affect us. We respect one another, and the hours we put in to save the lives of these majestic, stubborn, difficult dogs.

Helping rehome these dogs is one of the most gratifying things I do with my time. It's collaborative and challenging, and when you make the perfect placement, you feel as if you've done something meaningful. And here's a surprise: it's *meaning* that makes us happy, not a two-thousand-dollar Peloton.

Am I saying something as cornball as get your ass out from in front of your computer and go volunteer? Yeah, I am.

When I began writing this book, I thought there was a way to avoid the capitalistic consumer pressures to fritter away our limited resources trying to improve ourselves, without having to alter our online habits. I believed I was being realistic. And this book is about nothing if it's not about being realistic. What's the harm, if that's how we want to spend our precious time? The time is ours to waste, if we want to. I am, in fact, pro wasting time. I believed that despite the dozens of times a day we popped onto Instagram for a quick scroll, plummeting down the rabbit hole of the fantasies of other people's lives, we could still pay heed, the first and necessary step in knowing how and what to say yes to. We could be bilingual, as it were, fluent in losing ourselves for hours on the internet, while also speaking the old language of real-world experiences that bring us genuine joy and a sense of who we are.

But to say yes to the glories and mysteries of our human natures, to have a prayer of figuring out who we are and how to spend our time wisely, we must rethink our social media habit. I resisted coming to this conclusion for a long time. I was always the person at happy hour who ordered another round of margaritas while arguing that the internet is merely the Gutenberg printing press of our time, pass the chips and salsa please. The only thing I knew about the Gutenberg press was that it came along in the fifteenth century and allowed for the mass printing of books. I was pretty sure there were naysayers, just as there were about the rise of the internet. My argument was as unoriginal as it was inaccurate, that just because there will always be technological advances, all technological advances carry the same weight.

We've all been turned on to great stuff online. I've discovered new authors, TV shows, movies, and music I never would have known about otherwise. Podcasts in French, stylish yet comfy pants to wear on long-haul flights, a superb recipe for pie crust—all life-enriching goodies that have come my way because of the internet. But the question we need to ask ourselves is whether that's *enough*, given how the whole experience messes with our sense of self. Getting out now—by which I mean drastically reducing your time spent on social media—isn't the worst idea, and not just because life is easier and more enjoyable when we're not stuffing ourselves with images that trigger our compulsion to improve ourselves.

Deleting our social media accounts is unrealistic. We're too far down the road, and there are too many things, good things, that we love about the whole scene. It really has connected us to friends and family in a way that wasn't possible before. The rise of the gig economy has dovetailed nicely with the rise of tech—every freelancer, consultant, and small business needs a social media presence, or at least a website that links to it. It's here to stay, but we don't have to be enslaved to it. Breaking the habit of mindlessly picking up your phone to check likes etc. is the first and best thing you can do to reclaim your sense of self and your ability to know what is worth your time, energy, and focus.

Speaking of disengaging from the internet, let's not forget our daughters. Their habits are not yet formed. If you have a twelve-year-old with a smartphone, go tear that thing out of her hand right now. Rip out the battery and smash it to bits as if you're a kidnapper and you've caught the hostage trying to order an Uber. She will hate you, but chances are she already does anyway. Which is as it should be.

My husband and I save up our episodes of *Real Time with Bill Maher*, and when the day's gone to crap and we really feel like yelling at the TV we mix up some margaritas and settle in to watch. Recently, one of Bill's guests was social psychologist Jonathan Haidt, who's coauthored a book called *The Coddling of the American Mind: How Good Intentions and Bad Ideas Are Setting Up a Generation for Failure*. At first, it was the usual thing: kids today! What are ya gonna do? They're spoiled. They're entitled. They're the new Me Generation. Nothing we haven't heard before.

Then the subject turned to the disastrous effect of social media and smartphones on preteens. When boys get smartphones, they play video games and search for porn. When girls get smartphones, they post pictures of themselves and wait for the likes to pour in. Or not. As a result, the rates of anxiety, depression, and self-cutting have risen drastically. Suicide rates of young girls have gone up by 70 percent since 2009, the year when smartphones became all but ubiquitous.

In a September 2017 article in the *Guardian* entitled "You Are Your Looks: That's What Society Tells Girls. No Wonder They're Depressed," mental health activist Natasha Devon cites studies finding that girls as young as seven believe their appearance is the most important thing about them, and that stereotypes convince them "first that an ever more demanding paradigm of physical 'perfection' must be met with apparent effortlessness and then that being 'popular'—meek yet sociable—sexy but not 'slutty,' sporty in a narrow, feminine parameter (not 'too muscular') are imperatives."

The longer we keep our girls away from that shit the better. Every day a girl spends making collages or learning to draw or killing it on the soccer field or riding her skateboard, she is adding another wooden block in the Jenga game of her character. She's figuring out just a smidge more who she is, and in doing so, what she will find to be intolerable when it comes to "self-improvement." The more time we give our girls to figure out who their True Selves are, the greater the chance they'll be able to say yeah, no, not happening.

To engage in endless self-improvement is to continue to participate in a game that's rigged against us. As I write this, we're celebrating the one hundredth anniversary of women's suffrage. Movement leaders Susan B. Anthony and Elizabeth Cady Stanton gave their lives for the cause, which began to take shape in 1848.

Seventy-two years later, the Nineteenth Amendment was ratified by Congress, and it wasn't because they'd all just gotten laid and were in an exceptionally good mood. Generations of women have fought for our freedom to own property, to keep our jobs even though we are pregnant, to open bank accounts and apply for credit in our own names, to control our bodies and reproduction. It's been a two-steps-forward, one-step-back affair, but historically we have more rights than our mothers. This is not nothing.

That said, men and the systems they've built still rule. Look no further than the outcome of the 2016 American presidential election. Politics aside, one of the world's most powerful nations preferred the unqualified candidate with testicles to the candidate with more experience for the job than possibly anyone alive, who happened to be a woman. The oceans of ink, the miles of tweets and posts analyzing, interpreting, rationalizing, and finger-pointing change nothing. Of the 146 countries in the world, in 2017 only 15 were led by women, 8 of whom were the first female to hold that office. *Forbes*'s 2019 list of billionaires comprises mostly men; the richest woman in the world, ranked number fifteen, is Françoise Bettencourt Meyers, the granddaughter of the founder of L'Oréal cosmetics. How fitting.

"Humanity is male, and man defines woman," wrote Simone de Beauvoir in *The Second Sex*. And how does the patriarchy define us women, mostly? As humans who give birth, do for them, and buy stuff.

Women—we—and all the crap we buy and money we spend to improve ourselves throughout our lifetimes keep the economy that enriches mostly men afloat. We make cosmetic companies billions of dollars every year (see above). We support the luxe lives of plastic surgeons who specialize in keeping our faces, tummies, and vaginas forever young. We make motivational speakers and FLEBs multimillionaires and are the bread and butter of a cavalcade of micro-influencers. Together they create a mighty army of people with a vested interest in continuously moving the goalposts of self-improvery.

Corporations spend billions every year keeping women feeling insecure about every molecule of their being, and thus inclined to spend their hard-earned money on fixing what will prove to be unfixable. If the distressing condition *is* fixable, it will very soon go out of style/prove to be bad for your health/be not that important to your likability and fuckability, and it will be on to the next thing. Society becomes accepting of mothers who work, or women who want to stay home with their children, or women who don't want children, or women who without shame acknowledge and act on their own sex drive, or *whatever*—pick your freedom—and in a hot minute the "lifestyle" requires buying stuff and doing stuff to ensure we live it successfully.

The upshot is this: women may never be able to self-improve themselves out of their important role as Ms. Consumer. "Money gives men the power to run the show," said Beyoncé in 2013. "It gives the men power to define value. They define what's sexy. And men define what's feminine." The feminine ideal, defined by men, chased by women, forever and ever, amen.

We also cannot self-improve our way out of sexism and misogyny. We may be partnered with absolutely lovely men, but wait for one of those once-in-a-decade plate-smashing arguments and you might glimpse his essential feelings about women. We've established that he is a good man—the best!—but underneath his decency and kindness and impeccable socialization rests *his* short history of self-improvement during the late modern age involving the men who came before him, and how they felt about and related to women. Fathers who never learned how to operate the washing machine because it was beneath them. Grandfathers who treated their wives as if they were only slightly smarter than the family dog.

From 2004 to 2013 I wrote a rather lame monthly self-help column for *Redbook* magazine, and the number one question revolved around housework and why he wasn't doing his share. My advice seekers had tried everything, couples therapy and chore wheels and blow jobs in exchange for scrubbing the bathroom grout, but nothing worked for long. "Every time he changes a light bulb without being asked, he thinks he deserves the Congressional Medal of Honor," fumed one writer. Much thought has been given to this cosmic mystery. Do men just not *see* what needs to be done? Do they see it but don't believe it's an important use of their time? Do they see it and believe it's a good use of their time but just don't wanna? More likely, it's what my ex-husband hollered at me during one of the aforementioned plate-smashing arguments, "You should be doing it." Never mind that at the time I was also supporting the family.

In 1976, psychologist, scholar, and activist Dorothy Dinnerstein wrote a book called *The Mermaid and the Minotaur*, in which she posited that a host of domestic and political difficulties could be resolved if men shared equally in child-rearing. None of this "babysitting" his own kids or feeling like a good guy because he was helping their mother. If, in his heart, a father believed he was equally responsible for the care and upbringing of his children, it would change the way all men viewed women.

The cockroach-resiliency of the patriarchy exists, according to Dinnerstein, for the simple reason that psychologically men never quite recover from having been born of woman, then raised by her. Mom was the first and ultimate authority figure. Every moment of joy or sadness was in her control. He was coddled and smothered by her love. Or, he was criticized and humiliated by her. Most likely it was a combination of both because mothers are only human, trying to do their best. But no matter. Because a man's mother had all the power in his childhood, his unconscious holds her responsible for everything that sucks in his adult life. Dinnerstein believed that until fathers shared equally in the joy, burden, responsibility, *and* power of their parental role, boys would always possess the same "buried foundations" that prevent them from seeing males and females as equal.

Bottom line, we can't win if we play the game according to their rules.

The system may not be built for us, but we are, for the most part, freer than ever to operate inside of it. Running after the ever-receding mirage of ideal womanhood will never gain us the love, acceptance, and happiness that we seek. It's not de-signed to. But we're far from powerless. We can say yeah, no, not happening.

Why be the cash cow for the consumer economy? Why be-lieve the propaganda that only by trying to squeeze yourself into the culturally sanctioned cool-girl mold you are worthy of love? Why assume that someone on Instagram knows more about what's good for you than you do?

Why not save your money? Money is power.*

Why not pursue your cockamamie interests? Passions make life interesting. They give life meaning. Added bonus, they make *you* more interesting, both to yourself and to others.

Why not coax some of your repressed character traits out of the shadows and see what they're all about? The puritanism of self-improvement is so god-awful boring. It's not the worst thing in the world to knock back some cheap scotch and *skip yoga*.

I'm not suggesting you say fuck it all to everything—you will have to pry my bottle of Chanel No. 19 from my cold dead hands—just the bullshit that stresses you out, wastes your time, money, and energy, and promotes self-doubt and erodes self-trust. Life is a one-way turnstile. Time is our most precious commodity.

And if you still worry that saying yes to your True Self will

---

* Said Katharine Hepburn: "If you're given a choice between money and sex appeal, take the money. As you get older, the money will become your sex ap-peal."

make you unlovable, consider the story of Judith Taylor, an associate professor at the University of Toronto. One night in 2018 Professor Taylor was binge-watching *Friday Night Lights* and was struck by the character of Coach Eric Taylor, to whom she probably felt kinship, given they shared the same last name. How was it, she wondered, that Coach Taylor was considered by one and all to be a good guy, when he was also kind of a jerk? He was brusque, fair, firm, and took grief from no one. He bossed people around even when he was being supportive. He didn't bother connecting. Behavior, as we know, that is permitted in men but instantly renders women unlikable.

Professor Taylor was feeling overwhelmed by her workload at the time. She was the opposite of Coach Taylor, who issued orders and never offered an explanation. She worked hard to be kind and accommodating to her students, making sure they fully understood her reasoning behind each assignment and her grading decisions. Her door was always open.

She decided to run an experiment: what would happen if she traded in her identity as nice-as-pie Professor Taylor for the swaggering, always slightly pissed off Coach Taylor? Would her colleagues come to dislike her? Would her student evaluations suffer? Would she be shunned in the faculty lounge? Would she be written up by the dean?

For two weeks, she behaved like Coach Taylor. When students wandered into her office and mewled about the current assignment, asking if maybe they could do something *else*, she said, "Not gonna happen." The students shrugged, then did the original, objectionable assignment. Likewise, when a graduate student was dithering over her dissertation, she said, "Do you have what it takes? Then just do it."

"I came to meetings late," she wrote in a piece about her experiment in the *Toronto Star*. "I made jokes. Crucially, I started to meet colleagues for beers. . . . I was one of the only women, and my status was quickly elevated to one of the power brokers, and I joined the executive committee."

Her Coach Taylor strategy also worked at home. Over Sunday dinner she would say, "Here's how it's gonna go," and give her kids their chores for the week. They sort of looked at her like *what have you done with my mother*, but they cooperated.

In the end, Professor Taylor enjoyed success as Coach Taylor. Her students turned in more assignments, her kids complained less, and there was that promotion to the executive committee. She didn't much *like* herself that way, preferring to find a blend between cooperation, communication, and inclusivity, but our takeaway is this: no one hated her. Her husband didn't initiate divorce proceedings. Her kids went ahead and did what they were told, possibly glad for the structure. Her dean didn't discipline her. Nothing bad happened. No one stopped loving her, or even disliked her.

I'm not suggesting that if every woman in the world suddenly decided to embrace her inner asshole[*] there wouldn't be

---

[*] Excellent movie premise, however.

substantial pushback; rather, that deciding to stop being all things to all people all the time isn't always the personal calamity we imagine it might be. Despite the reality of the double bind, there's more room to maneuver than we suppose.

That said, when you're a young woman with your romantic and domestic future ahead of you, it takes courage to channel your inner Coach Taylor. In *Bitch Doctrine: Essays for Dissenting Adults*, British journalist and activist Laurie Penny writes about the real choices women in their twenties are often forced to make between being true to themselves and being partnered with dolts who are happy to sleep with them until they sense there's an actual person in there with interests, passions, opinions, and proclivities.

"Nothing frustrates me so much as watching young women at the start of their lives wasting years in succession on lackluster, unappreciative, boring child-men, who were only ever looking for a magic girl to show off to their friends, a girl who would in private be both surrogate mother and sex partner. I've been that girl. It's no fun being that girl."

Penny could never quite bring herself to be that girl. She would sleep with a guy for a month or more, then he would ghost. She was sad. Her heart was banged up if not broken. She grieved for a bit that she couldn't make herself more "stereotypically lovable."

"With hindsight, though, I'm glad that I've never been willing or able to narrow my horizons for a man. It didn't turn out to be half as scary, or a fraction as lonely, as I'd been told."

I'm not going to lie to you. It's a little dangerous to live a life in which you do what you want to do, behave in a way that feels authentic, pay attention to things you find of interest, and direct your passions in any way you see fit.

You are now a woman who can't be controlled by mass media and consumer culture.

Congratulations, sister.

In 1977 the great poet Adrienne Rich delivered a commencement speech at Douglass College, and her words remain distressingly relevant today, over forty years later. Douglass College, part of Rutgers University, was founded in 1918 as the New Jersey College for Women, and Rich's audience was all female. In her speech, she encouraged them to be aware that the education they've received reflects the male view of the world. That the so-called great issues and mainstream Western thought are their issues, their thoughts, excluding half of the population, excluding women. She seemed to have been leading into a talk about the importance of women's studies, but that was not her true concern. Her subject was the importance of responsibility for ourselves. She said, "Responsibility to yourself means that you don't fall for shallow and easy solutions—predigested books and ideas, weekend encounters guaranteed to change your life. . . . It means that you refuse to sell your talents and aspirations short, simply to avoid conflict and confrontation. And this, in turn, means resisting the forces in society which say that women should be nice, play safe, have low professional expectations, drown in love and forget about work, live through others, and stay in the places assigned to us."

It's time to say yeah, no, not happening. Because life is beautifully complicated and we are beautifully complicated, yet we would happily trade complexity for endless happiness, an impossible feat. Because we don't really know what makes us happy, because we've become less interested in knowing ourselves, and more interested in doing a new program that will make us like someone else. Because many young girls claim they would rather be blind than fat. Because their older sisters, cousins, aunts, and mothers would trade five years of their lives to be thin without having to diet. Because the colossal energy we direct toward endlessly improving ourselves could be spent on higher, more varied and interesting pursuits, not to mention improving our communities and the world at large. Because we watch beloved friends spend more and more of their precious days, their limited time, in the existential swamp of working toward a state that's impossible to attain. Because we watch our exquisite daughters forgo joy in the moment because they feel as if they don't deserve it but will at some future time when they become thinner, fitter, more organized, more productive, more positive, and sweeter. Because regardless of whether the pressure is cultural, societal, familial, or social media-al—it's time for all of us to say fuck it all to self-improvement. It's time to take back ourselves.

Epilogue: Collioure

... the only people for me are the mad ones, the ones who are mad to live, mad to talk, mad to be saved, desirous of everything at the same time, the ones who never yawn or say a commonplace thing, but burn, burn, burn like fabulous yellow roman candles exploding like spiders across the stars.

—Jack Kerouac, *On the Road*

After I lived with my True Self for a while, it occurred to me that more of my life was behind me rather than in front of me. While I was sitting with my mortality, I came upon one of the chestnuts of the internet, possibly the best one—Australian hospice nurse Bronnie Ware's 2009 blog post listing the top five most common regrets of the dying. The post garnered millions of views; by 2012 the number was eight million and counting. Ware then wrote a memoir called, fittingly, *The Top Five Regrets of the Dying*. It was translated into twenty-seven languages. The top regret was:

I wish I'd had the courage to live a life true to myself, not the life others expected of me.

We think we're taking ourselves and our lives seriously when we're immersed in optimizing every moment of every day, fine-tuning our already perfectly fine diet, weighing ourselves every morning long after we can no longer see the numbers on the scale without glasses, working, always working, to be better, to be best.

It's the longest con out there, self-improvement.

Thinking endlessly about self-improvement takes up a lot of headspace and time. Once you've sworn it off, you find yourself with a lot of room to think. At night, as I was drifting off to sleep, I thought of Bronnie Ware's elders, and how they regretted not having had the courage to be who they were. I would think: *I am as free as I will ever be.* My daughter is grown-up, my parents are both gone, I have a (very) little money in the bank. I thought about Mary Oliver's oft-quoted, yet still awesome, line: "What is it you plan to do with your one wild and precious life?"

I remembered something I hadn't thought of in decades: after my mother died, I found among her things a file labeled Dream Trip. It was stuffed with clippings of things to do in London, Vienna, Paris, and Rome. She was waiting to go. Waiting until I was launched. Waiting until money wasn't so tight. Waiting until my father could take off three weeks instead of the two he was allotted. There was always a perfectly good reason now was not the time to go. I remembered a moment with my mother, bloated and bald from chemo. She said, "I guess I will never get to Vienna." And then she died. She was forty-six.

The day after our daughter got married in June 2018, I decided I needed to turn the final card over and risk being who I believed myself to be: a woman who made her dream of living in France come true. We put our 102-year-old gray colonial with the straggly pink rose bushes up for sale, sold our old VW Cabrio, got rid of most of our stuff, and moved to a village named Collioure.

I am writing this to you from there.

Collioure is an ancient village on the Mediterranean, where the Pyrenees mountains meet the sea. It's most famous for being the place where Henri Matisse discovered his bright fauve palette. Before Collioure, Matisse was a traditionalist with a dwindling career; in 1905 he discovered the light of Collioure, the red-and-blue anchovy boats, the pink glow of sky and ocean at dusk, the deep green of the ancient vineyards blanketing the hillsides.

My husband and I live in a tiny apartment with stone walls and green wooden shutters with peeling paint, over the nougat shop and across from the second-rate boulangerie. We swim in the sea every day, and like Jenny Odell and her bird-watching, I have become a sea-watcher, attuning myself to its different moods depending on whether there had been a storm or what direction the wind is coming from. Sometimes the sea is smooth green glass; other times it's gray and disorganized. When the wind is in from Africa, everything in the village is covered in a fine ocher-colored dust. After our swim, we have a glass of local rosé at the St. Elme, our favorite seaside café.

Imperfection is an art here. Some days the boulangerie has enough croissants for its customers and sometimes it doesn't. The shops close for lunch, until whenever it suits them to open in the afternoon. There is an army barracks where the French commandos live while in training, and the French flag is raised anywhere between 7:20 and 8:00 a.m. each day. There is no such thing as on the dot, or ice-cold beer, or people who can't stop to have a tepid one with a friend. Every day I speak my B-minus level French, and hope that it will improve, but I'm not counting on it.

The French people I've met in our new home say yeah, no, not happening as if they were born to it. They say it with a smirk. Even if eventually they will say yes, and . . . they always start with no. It amuses them, I'm told, to be convinced to say yes. It allows for a conversation. As for self-improvement, they find it uninteresting. They prize originality and the willingness to see what happens next.

Notes

INTRODUCTION: HELLO YOU

xi   Created not by bison hunters: Three-quarters of hand stencils in eight caves in France and Spain were determined to be female, according to a study conducted by archeologist Dean Snow, under the auspices of *National Geographic*. Virginia Hughes, "Were the First Artists Mostly Women?" *National Geographic*, October 9, 2013.

xi   Then came the wealthy: Alastair Sooke, "How Ancient Egypt Shaped Our Idea of Beauty," BBC.com, February 4, 2016.

xi   Eleanor of Aquitaine, queen: Alison Weir, *Eleanor of Aquitaine* (New York: Ballantine Books, 2000).

xiii   One *Huffington Post* piece: Ester Bloom, "How 'Treat Yourself' Became a Capitalist Command," *Atlantic*, November 19, 2015.

xviii   There are over a thousand known varieties of bananas: "Banana Facts and Figures," Food and Agriculture Organization of the United Nations, 2018, fao.org/economic/est/est-commodities/bananas/bananafacts.

CHAPTER 1: TODAY IS THE DAY

8   Over the past decade microbiologists: M. Valles-Colomer, G. Falony, Y. Darzi, et al., "The Neuroactive Potential of the Human Gut Microbiota in Quality of Life and Depression," *Nature Microbiology*, February 2019.

8   unless you've participated in the American Gut Project: americangut.org.

13   The Voldemort of emotions: Brené Brown, *I Thought It Was Just Me (but it isn't): Making the Journey from "What Will People Think?" to "I Am Enough"* (New York: Avery, 2007), introduction.

14   Shame, as Brown defines: Brown, *I Thought It Was Just Me*, chapter 1.

17   During Brown's investigation: Brown, *I Thought It Was Just Me*, chapter 3.

17   during the last decade: Sharon M. Fruh et al., "Obesity Stigma and Bias," *Journal for Nurse Practitioners* 12, no. 7 (July–August 2016): 425–32.

18   A groundbreaking piece of research: Meghan L. Meyer and Matthew D. Lieberman, "Why People Are Always Thinking about Themselves: Medial Prefrontal Cortex Activity during Rest Primes Self-Referential Processing," *Journal of Cognitive Neuroscience* 30, no. 5 (May 2018): 714–21.

19   The growing sophistication of technology: Jessica R. Andrews-Hanna, "The Brain's Default Network and Its Adaptive Role in Internal Mentation," *Neuroscientist* 18, no. 3 (June 2012): 251–70.

CHAPTER 2: THE GREAT FEMALE SELF-IMPROVEMENT BAMBOOZLEMENT

22   Behold an advertisement in a 1919 issue of *Ladies' Home Journal*: Sarah Everts, "How Advertisers Convinced Americans They Smelled Bad," Smithsonian.com, August 2, 2012.

23   A 1923 ad campaign: Marlen Komar, "How One Everyday Beauty Product Is Responsible for the Most Outdated Marriage Cliche Ever," Bustle .com, July 12, 2017.

24   In 2018 women spent: Statista Research Department, "Total Consumer Spending of Women Worldwide in 2013 and 2018," Statista.com, August 9, 2019.

24   A 2015 article in *Forbes*: Bridget Brennan, "Top 10 Things Everyone Should Know About Women Consumers," *Forbes*, January 21, 2015.

24   As cultural critic Ellen Willis: Ellen Willis, "Women and the Myth of Consumerism," *Ramparts*, 8, no. 12 (June 1970): 13–16.

25   Enter the clever tactic: "History of Philip Morris," Center for Media and Democracy, SourceWatch.org, 1987, November 24, 2015.

26   Philip Morris also manufactured Virginia Slims: Centers for Disease Control and Prevention, "Women and Smoking: A Report of the Surgeon General," *MMWR* 51, no. RR-12 (August 2002).

27   A study published in: Debra Trampe, Diederik A. Stapel, and Frans W. Siero, "The Self-Activation Effect of Advertisements: Ads Can Affect Whether and How Consumers Think About the Self," *Journal of Consumer Research* 37, no. 6 (April 2011). (Note: It has since been retracted.)

32   She may have said: Simone de Beauvoir, *The Coming of Age*, reprint edition (New York: W. W. Norton & Company, 1996), conclusion.

34   As I write this: Todd Spangler, "Are Americans Addicted to Smartphones? U.S. Consumers Check Their Phones 52 Times Daily, Study Finds," *Variety*, November 14, 2018.

36   Will Storr, writing in: Will Storr, *Selfie: How We Became So Self-Obsessed and What It's Doing to Us* (New York: Harry N. Abrams, 2018), book zero.

38   They practice something Canadian writer: Kelly Diels, "Female Lifestyle Empowerment Brand," kellydiels.com.

39   Vox reported in 2018: Julia Belluz, "Goop Was Fined $145,000 for Its Claims about Jade Eggs for Vaginas. It's Still Selling Them," Vox.com, September 6, 2018.

42   Carina Chocano, author of: Carina Chocano, "The Coast of Utopia," *Vanity Fair*, August 2019.

44   Look no further than: Hayley Krischer, "The New Mom Uniform of Park Slope," *New York Times*, January 16, 2019.

44   Pioneered by twentieth-century French philosopher: René Girard, *Deceit, Desire, and the Novel: Self and Other in Literary Structure* (Baltimore: Johns Hopkins University Press, 1976).

CHAPTER 3: IT'S COMPLICATED: SELF-IMPROVEMENT FOR GIRLS

51   I could "watch my figure": Ellen Peck, *How to Get a Teen-Age Boy and What to Do with Him When You Get Him* (New York: Bernard Geis Associates, 1969). You really can't make this stuff up.

55   In *Kids These Days*: Malcolm Harris, *Kids These Days: Human Capital and the Making of Millennials* (New York: Little, Brown and Company, 2017), chapter 3.

55   One of the fallouts: "Billionaire Fortunes Grew by $2.5 Billion a Day Last Year as Poorest Saw Their Wealth Fall," Oxfam International, January 21, 2019, https://www.oxfam.org/en/press-releases/billionaire-fortunes-grew-25-billion-day-last-year-poorest-saw-their-wealth-fall.

56   A January 2019 article: Adam Schubak, "20 Ways to Be the Best You in 2019," *Men's Health*, January 9, 2019.

57   Let us never forget: Eugene Scott, "White Women Helped Elect Trump. Now He's Losing Their Support," *Washington Post*, January 22, 2018.

60   In 2008, candidate Mitt Romney: Morgan Little, "Mitt, Ann Romney Defend Putting Dog on Car Roof; Fallout Continues," *Los Angeles Times*, April 17, 2012.

61   Joan C. Williams, in: Joan C. Williams, "How Women Can Escape the Likability Trap: Powerful Women Know How to Flip Feminine Stereotypes to Their Advantage," *New York Times*, August 16, 2019.

64   Jia Tolentino, writing about: Jia Tolentino, *Trick Mirror: Reflections on Self-Delusion* (New York: Random House, 2019), 78.

CHAPTER 4: YOUR BEST SELF IS LIKE AN IMAGINARY BELOVED

70   One contributor to Thought Catalog: Claudia St. Claire, "I Have an Imaginary Boyfriend," Thought Catalog, January 21, 2014.

71   Second-wave feminism effectively: Laura Mulvey, "Visual Pleasure and Narrative Cinema," *Screen*, Autumn 1975.

72   "A woman must continually": John Berger, *Ways of Seeing: Based on the BBC Television Series*, reprint edition (New York: Penguin Books, 1990), 46.

74   Kathryn Schulz, writing in: Kathryn Schulz, "The Self in Self-Help," *New York* magazine, January 4, 2013.

75   Those who suffer from: Katharine A. Phillips et al., "Body Dysmorphic Disorder: Some Key Issues for DSM-V," *Depression and Anxiety* 27, no. 6 (June 2010): 573–91.

CHAPTER 5: A SHORT HISTORY OF SELF-IMPROVEMENT DURING THE LATE MODERN AGE

93   Then new machine technologies: Stephen Nicholas and Deborah Oxley, "The Living Standards of Women during the Industrial Revolution, 1795–1820," *Economic History Review* 46, no. 4 (November 1993): 723–49.

94   At the end of the nineteenth century: Francis Parkman, "The Woman Question," *North American Review* 129, no. 275 (October 1879): 303–21.

94   English philosopher John Locke: Helena Rodrigues, "In Defense of Women: Equality in Locke's Political Theory" (The Midwest Political Science Association, Palmer House Hilton, Chicago, Illinois, April 15, 2004).

95   A generation later French writer: Jean-Jacques Rousseau, *Emile, or On Education* (New York: Penguin Classics, 2007), Book V.

99   Symptoms included insomnia, anxiety: Rachel P. Maines, *The Technology of Orgasm: "Hysteria," the Vibrator, and Women's Sexual Satisfaction* (Baltimore: Johns Hopkins University Press, 1999), chapter 1.

99   Psychologist and educator G. Stanley Hall: G. Stanley Hall, *Adolescence*, Vol. II (New York: D. Appleton, 1905), 588.

100   It is as if the Almighty: Ann Douglas Wood, "The 'Fashionable Diseases': Women's Complaints and Their Treatment in Nineteenth-Century America," *Journal of Interdisciplinary History* 4 (Summer 1973): 29.

100   He believed the ovaries: Rita Arditti, "Women as Objects: Science and Sexual Politics," Science for the People, September 1974, 8.

100   By 1906, 150,000 women: Ehrenreich and English, 136.

103   Ellen Swallow Richards, the founder: Barbara Ehrenreich and Deirdre English, *For Her Own Good: Two Centuries of the Experts' Advice to Women*, rev. ed. (New York: Anchor Books, 2005), chapter 5.

108   Around the same: Susan Contratto, "Psychology Views Mothers and Mothering: 1897–1980," *Feminist Re-visions: What Has Been and Might Be* (Ann Arbor: University of Michigan, 1983).

109   His theory, developed: Ibid.

110   In 1963, she published: Stephanie Coontz, *A Strange Stirring: The Feminine Mystique and American Women at the Dawn of the 1960s* (New York: Basic Books, 2011), chapter 8.

112   Helen Gurley was one: Brooke Hauser, *Enter Helen: The Invention of Helen Gurley Brown and the Rise of the Modern Single Woman* (New York: Harper, 2016).

113   She is demonstrating: Nora Ephron, "Helen Gurley Brown: 'If You're a Little Mouseburger, Come with Me. I Was a Mouseburger and I Can Help You.' *The Most of Nora Ephron* (New York: Knopf, 2013), 86.

115   By 1980, half: George Guilder, "Women in the Work Force," *Atlantic*, September 1986.

116   It was 1982, and: Jennifer Szalai, "The Complicated Origins of 'Having It All,'" *New York Times Magazine*, January 2, 2015.

CHAPTER 6: WHERE THE WILD THINGS STILL ARE

123   Mark Manson, the King: Mark Manson, "The Staggering Bullshit of 'The Secret,'" MarkManson.net.

127   These books take: Sadie Trombetta, "Women Are Angrier Than Ever, and These 3 Books Explore What That Means," Bustle, September 27, 2018.

128   Which brings us to: Carl Jung, "Aion: Phenomenology of the Self," in Joseph Campbell (ed.), *The Portable Jung* (New York: The Viking Press, 1971).

CHAPTER 7: TRUE YOU RISING

143   I read a little: Ralph Waldo Emerson, *Emerson: Essays and Lectures* (New York: Library of America, 1983), 1107.

149   Writing in the *Los Angeles Times*: Jennifer Conlin, "The $10-Billion Business of Self-Care," *Los Angeles Times*, May 10, 2019.

150   According to Samsung: Rachel Jacoby Zoldan, "This Is the Estimated Number of Selfies You'll Take in a Lifetime," *Teen Vogue*, March 31, 2017.

151   Stein lived in Paris: Gertrude Stein, *The Autobiography of Alice B. Toklas*, reissue edition (New York: Vintage, 1990).

CHAPTER 8: THE YEAH, NO. NOT HAPPENING CHEAT SHEET

162   But there were: Soraya Nadia McDonald, "Kim Novak Responds to Post-Oscars Ridicule: 'I Was Bullied,'" *Washington Post*, April 18, 2014.

164   In 2006, Duke: Yang Yang, "On the Dynamics of, and Heterogeneity in, Subjective Well-Being Across the Life Course and Over Time in the United States," *SINET*, May & August no. 94 & 95 (2008).

166   Jessica Valenti sums: Jessica Valenti, "She Who Dies with the Most 'Likes' Wins?" *Nation*, November 29, 2012.

171   In *Secrets from*: Traci Mann, *Secrets from the Eating Lab: The Science of Weight Loss, the Myth of Willpower, and Why You Should Never Diet Again* (New York: Harper Wave, 2015), chapter 2.

176   From *Parents* magazine: Lauren Wiener, "Stressed? 28 Ways to Unwind—By Tonight!" *Parents*, undated.

CHAPTER 9: WHY YES, AND . . .

186   Stanford professor emerita: Patricia Ryan Madson, *Improv Wisdom: Don't Prepare, Just Show Up* (New York: Bell Tower, 2005).

189   Based in Oakland: Jenny Odell, "How to Do Nothing," Medium.com, June 29, 2017.

190   "When I go biking, I repeat," *A Natural History of the Senses* (New York: Vintage, 1991), 184.

200   "Money gives men power": Noreen Malone, "Can Women Have It All? Beyoncé Says Yes," *New Republic*, January 27, 2013.

202   The cockroach-resiliency: Dorothy Dinnerstein, *The Mermaid and the Minotaur: Sexual Arrangements and Human Malaise* (New York: Harper & Row, 1976; repr. New York: Other Press, 1999).

205   "I came to meetings": Judith Taylor, "I'm a woman who imitated the swagger of an entitled white male—and it got results," *The Star*, October 13, 2018.

206   "Nothing frustrates me so": Laurie Penny, *Bitch Doctrine: Essays for Dissenting Adults* (New York: Bloomsbury, 2017).

207   "Responsibility to yourself": Adrienne Rich, "Claiming an Education," *On Lies, Secrets, and Silence: Selected Prose 1966–1978* (New York: W.W. Norton, 1979), 233–234.

About the Author

KAREN KARBO is the author of *Trespassers Welcome Here*, *The Diamond Lane*, and *Motherhood Made a Man Out of Me*; the memoir *The Stuff of Life*; and the Kick Ass Women series. Her short stories, essays, articles, and reviews have appeared in numerous publications, including the *New York Times*. She is a recipient of a National Endowment for the Arts Fellowship in Fiction and a winner of the General Electric Younger Writer Award. In addition, Karbo penned three books in the Minerva Clark mystery series for children. A longtime resident of Portland, Oregon, she now lives in Collioure, France.